COACHING COLLEGE STUDENTS
WITH EXECUTIVE FUNCTION PROBLEMS

Coaching
College Students
with Executive Function
Problems

Mary R. T. Kennedy

Foreword by McKay Moore Sohlberg

THE GUILFORD PRESS
New York   London

The author has checked with sources believed to be reliable in her efforts to provide information
that is complete and generally in accord with the standards of practice that are accepted at the time
of publication. However, in view of the possibility of human error or changes in behavioral, mental
health, or medical sciences, neither the author, nor the editors and publisher, nor any other party
who has been involved in the preparation or publication of this work warrants that the information
contained herein is in every respect accurate or complete, and they are not responsible for any errors
or omissions or the results obtained from the use of such information. Readers are encouraged to
confirm the information contained in this book with other sources.

Library of Congress Cataloging-in-Publication Data

Names: Kennedy, Mary R. T., author.
Title: Coaching college students with executive function problems / Mary R.T.
    Kennedy.
Description: New York : Guilford Press, [2017] | Includes bibliographical
    references and index.
Identifiers: LCCN 2016052192 | ISBN 9781462531332 (pbk. : acid-free paper)
Subjects: LCSH: Learning disabled—Education (Higher) | People with mental
    disabilities—Education (Higher) | College students with
    disabilities—Services for. | Executive functions (Neuropsychology) |
    Mentoring in education.
Classification: LCC LC4818.38 .K46 2017 | DDC 378.0087—dc23
LC record available at https://lccn.loc.gov/2016052192

To my husband, Paul Kennedy; my mom, Betty Thompson;
and my daughter, Erin Trudeau.
Your love and support sustained me through this long process.

And in memory of my dad, Corry Thompson,
for his passion of a college education for all individuals.

About the Author

Mary R. T. Kennedy, PhD, CCC-SLP, is Professor and Chair of the Department of Communication Sciences and Disorders at Chapman University in Orange, California. She is a certified speech–language pathologist who has worked with individuals with acquired brain injury for many years. Board certified by the Academy of Neurologic Communication Disorders and Sciences (ANCDS), Dr. Kennedy is a Fellow of the American Speech–Language–Hearing Association and a recipient of the ANCDS Honors Award. She has been associate editor and guest editor for peer-reviewed journals on topics related to brain injury. Dr. Kennedy's research and more than 60 publications have focused on management of cognitive and language disorders after brain injury. Her current work documents common challenges facing college students with brain injury, and validates the usefulness of coaching that explicitly instructs students in self-regulation so as to support executive functions.

Foreword

It is very exciting to be writing a foreword to a book dedicated to assisting students who struggle in college owing to challenges with executive functions. Not so long ago, this book simply would have had no audience. The prevailing belief was that the populations discussed in the book, particularly students with brain injury, could not successfully pursue a college degree. Today we know better.

The Americans with Disabilities Act (passed in 1990, with subsequent amendments in 2008) promulgated regulations to make education accessible to students with learning difficulties. As a result, substantial numbers of students who have either executive function deficits or an acquired neurological insult are now enrolled in postsecondary education. According to the Council for Learning Disabilities, postsecondary education is now the goal of 80% of students with disabilities. Legal protections, thankfully, are in place.

Ensuring that these students can matriculate is the first critical step in safeguarding their right to a college education. The next step is to ensure that these students receive adequate supports while attending college. Disability services offices exist on most college and university campuses and are responsible for providing these intensive supports. However, in spite of this growing need, diminished funding for these educational resources precludes these offices from fulfilling their role. Unfortunately, blanket classroom accommodations are an all-too-common response. The structure provided by the dynamic coaching model described in *Coaching College Students with Executive Function Problems* is an option that can be incorporated into support services and, when necessary, integrated with individualized accommodations. This coaching model contains clear protocols that enable it to be delivered by coaches from a wide variety of professional backgrounds, making it adaptable for different support service contexts. Because dynamic coaching steers students toward self-management, the model has the added benefit of requiring fewer supports over time. By following the book's tenets, coaches can effectively help students who struggle with executive functions to acquire the skills necessary to self-advocate, and can teach them to generate, initiate, and evaluate self-selected strategies to meet their own academic goals. In so doing, students' executive functions improve.

During the period of increased legislative advocacy for students with cognitive challenges, there has been a commensurate growth in our understanding of the underlying mechanisms of their challenges and in the processes that can lead to improved functioning. *Coaching College Students with Executive Function Problems* reflects our expanded knowledge in a number of domains in cognitive psychology. We now have a deeper understanding of the nature of executive functions as a complex multicomponent system, which is also interdependent on other cognitive networks. In particular, our increased knowledge of how metacognition serves learning and task execution, elucidated through the expansive work conducted by Kennedy and others, has helped us to appreciate the preeminent role these superordinate processes play in our functional abilities, especially the abilities needed for successful learning. Teaching students with executive function challenges to evaluate their own performance in relation to the strategies they initiate leverages the metacognitive skills necessary for ongoing self-management in school, and, in turn, improves students' executive functions.

Our deeper understanding of the importance of self-determination in learning is also reflected in the model prescribed in this book. Self-determination includes the sense of autonomy, or the sense that our own actions are self-endorsed and consistent with our own values and interests. The dynamic coaching model is based on the student identifying his or her needs and goals. The student drives the intervention. Self-determination also relies on a sense of competence or belief that we can successfully implement a skill or action. This ability, often referred to as self-efficacy, is at the heart of dynamic coaching. The iterative cycle of self-evaluation and refinement of strategies and goals reinforces self-determination.

Another arena critical to clinical advancement is that of therapeutic alliance. While the concept of therapeutic alliance is not new, the application of therapeutic alliance to working with people who have cognitive deficits has not been part of mainstream therapy. In recent years, we have begun to realize the power that the relationship between therapists and clients has in helping our clients optimize their response to treatment or coaching. Most models of therapeutic alliance include aspects of these three elements: agreement about the goals being addressed, agreement about the tasks to address the goals, and a personal bond made up of reciprocal feelings. Motivational interviewing, detailed in this book, is one model that incorporates these elements, and consists of an important set of skills that the reader is encouraged to study closely.

In short, the dynamic coaching processes advocated in this book integrate the active ingredients of metacognitive strategy training, instilling self-determination, and creating a therapeutic alliance into an intervention model that is feasible to implement. Other books offer descriptions and explanations of conditions and therapeutic responses, but lack the scaffolding to make implementation possible. Kennedy does not just tell us *what* to do as clinicians or coaches, she also tells us *how* to do it, and provides us with protocols to make it happen.

Coaching College Students with Executive Function Problems is more than a checklist of teaching activities; it is a resource that provides professionals an evidence-based road map to ensure that their students are successful. However, it is the reader's task to learn and embrace the processes and techniques. Working with the students using the dynamic coaching model requires a commitment and a coaching mindset. While Kennedy has manualized the approach and explained the components, ultimately, it is the coach's responsibility to honor the relational nature of the training. Effective implementation requires that coaches focus less on viewing themselves as experts who deliver treatment and more on empowering students to become equal partners in collaborating on finding solutions to their problems. Supported by a strong research foundation, the methods are effective for helping students with executive function problems learn to successfully self-manage in school. The processes are also rewarding and fulfilling for both partners in the coaching dyad—the student and the coach—to implement.

MCKAY MOORE SOHLBERG, PhD
HEDCO Professor
Communication Disorders and Sciences
College of Education, University of Oregon

Acknowledgments

Huge thanks to the clinician-coaches Miriam Krause, PhD, CCC-SLP, Katy H. O'Brien, PhD, CCC-SLP, and Sarah Schellinger, PhD, CCC-SLP—especially to you, Katy, for the many hours we spent at coffee shops talking about and creating the work represented in this book! My own thinking about coaching and how it is described in this book would not have been possible without the countless discussions of our coaching practices.

To graduate students Gina DeSalvio and Monica Gannon: Thank you for keeping all of the pieces organized, referenced, and formatted. I could not have done it without you!

To the college students with brain injury: You inspired me to figure out how to help you navigate your own way through college.

And a special acknowledgment to Rochelle Serwator, my editor at The Guilford Press, for being so understanding, encouraging, and supportive over the past few years.

Contents

List of Figures, Forms, and Tables   xv

Introduction   1

PART I. FOUNDATIONS

1. Executive Functions and Self-Regulation   7
   What Are Executive Functions?   8
   What Is Self-Regulation and How Is It Related to Executive Functions?   15

2. College Students with Executive Function Problems   22
   College Students with Developmental Disabilities and Executive Function Problems   25
   College Students with Acquired Brain Injury and Executive Function Problems   28
   APPENDIX 2.1. What Disability Service Specialists Should Know about Concussion   33

3. Military Service Members and Veterans in College   37
   Donald L. MacLennan and Leslie Nitta

   Blasts, TBI, and the Wounds of War   37
   Considering the Military Culture in an Educational Context   43
   A Summary of Recommendations for Postsecondary Settings   52
   Additional Resources   53

PART II. DYNAMIC COACHING

4. A Dynamic Coaching Approach   57
   Who Are Dynamic Coaches?   58
   Models for Coaching Students in Executive Functions   58

A Dynamic Approach to Coaching Self-Regulation   62
Student Benefits Associated with Coaching   79
Additional Resources   82

5. Information Gathering and Collaborative Planning   92
Questionnaires, Interviews, and Tests   93
Collaborative Planning: Translation, Goal Writing, Student Outcomes,
    and Individualized Plans   107

6. Coaching Self-Management and Self-Learning: 159
Goals—Strategies—Act—Adjust
with Katy H. O'Brien
Goal Setting in Self-Learning   162
Goal Setting in Self-Management   166
Strategizing for Self-Learning   170
Strategizing for Self-Management   174
Managing Ineffective Strategies   182
Taking Action: Tracking Strategies and Performance in Self-Learning
    and Self-Management   184
Adjustment: Strategy Usefulness and Next Steps   186
Additional Resources   188

7. Coaching Self-Advocacy   190
What Coaches Need to Know about Self-Advocacy in College Students   191
Student Rights, Responsibilities, and Self-Advocacy Skills   195
Coaching Self-Advocacy Using the GSAA Approach   198
Additional Resources   210

8. Coaching toward Independence   212
Tools That Foster Self-Coaching   212
Integrating Dynamic Coaching into Your Practice   214

References   217

Index   233

List of Figures, Forms, and Tables

FIGURES

FIGURE 1.1. Model of self-regulation. 16

FIGURE 2.1. The percentage of postsecondary institutions that enrolled 23
college students with disability by category from the NCES report.

FIGURE 2.2. The percentage of students by disability categories 24
at postsecondary institutions from the NCES report.

FIGURE 2.3. Three domains of symptoms that interact and overlap 31
after a concussion.

FIGURE 4.1. Phases of coaching. 68

FIGURE 4.2. The self-regulation process in steps. 74

FIGURE 5.1. A flowchart of information-gathering components 94
and steps for coaches to follow.

FIGURE 5.2. Examples of mapping proximal and distal goals onto a plan 116
by immediacy of need.

FIGURE 5.3. Sample self-regulation goals to pair with proximal goals. 117

FIGURE 6.1. Sample scaled self-learning goal using GAS. 164

FIGURE 6.2. Action-Planning Form (Form 4.6) for a student 165
with memory impairments.

FIGURE 7.1.   The percentage of postsecondary institutions that provide   197
              these specific accommodations to college students.

FIGURE 7.2.   A sample of how to create a team   202
              using the Action-Planning Form (Form 4.6).

FIGURE 7.3.   Taking an exam in the disability services center   206
              using the Action-Planning Form (Form 4.6).

FORMS

FORM 4.1.   What to Expect with Dynamic Coaching   83

FORM 4.2.   Self-Reflection: Start   84

FORM 4.3.   Self-Reflection: End   85

FORM 4.4.   Tracking Strategy Action   86

FORM 4.5.   Strategy Usefulness and Next Steps   87

FORM 4.6.   Action-Planning Form   88

FORM 4.7.   Student Summary of Strategies   90

FORM 4.8.   Strategy Review and Other Applications   91

FORM 5.1.   Getting Started Checklist for Coaches   119

FORM 5.2.   Getting Started Checklist for Students   120

FORM 5.3.   Demographic, Academic, Medical, and Social History Form   121

FORM 5.4.   College Survey for Students with Other Disabilities (CSS-OD)   125

FORM 5.5.   College Survey for Students with Brain Injury (CSS-BI)   130

FORM 5.6.   College Survey for Students with Concussion (CSS-C)   136

FORM 5.7.   Academic Statements from the CSS-OD, CSS-BI,   143
             and CSS-C, with Importance Ratings and Follow-Up Questions

FORM 5.8.   Interpreting Abilities and Disabilities   149

FORM 5.9.   Templates for Goal Attainment Scaling   151

FORM 5.10.   A List of Goals by Immediacy, Ranging from Weeks to Years   156

FORM 5.11.   Mapping Proximal and Distal Goals onto a Plan by Immediacy of Need   157

FORM 6.1.   Plan–Do–Review   189

FORM 7.1.   Team Members   211

TABLES

TABLE 1.1.   Cognitive, Language, Physical, and Sensory Processes   9
and How Impairments in These Domains May Manifest in Students'
Ability to Succeed Academically and Socially in College

TABLE 1.2.   Executive Functions and How Impairments in These Domains   13
May Be Manifest in Students' Abilities in College

TABLE 3.1.   Aspects of Battlemind and How These Aspects Relate   44
to the College Experiences of Service Member and Veteran Students

TABLE 4.1.   Stages of Change and Complementary Coaching Strategies   60
for Students with Executive Function Problems

TABLE 4.2.   MI Questions (OARS) and Examples That Could Be Used   65
When Coaching Students Through Complex Situations

TABLE 4.3.   What Good Coaches Do and Do Not Do   67

TABLE 4.4.   Similarities and Differences between Dynamic Coaching   78
and Didactic Instruction

TABLE 5.1.   Surveys, Questionnaires, and Tests for Evaluating College Students   99
with Executive Function Problems, Listed Alphabetically

TABLE 5.2.   Using Students' Academic Challenges from the College Survey   104
to Ask Deeper Questions about Strategies
in a Semistructured Interview

TABLE 5.3.   Examples of How Self-Regulation and Performance Goals   111
Are Generated and Are Related to Each Other

TABLE 6.1.   Sample Goal Development for Studying and Learning   163

TABLE 6.2.   Sample Goal Development for Time Management   169

TABLE 6.3.   Studying, Learning, and Memory Techniques That Include   171
Aspects of Self-Regulation

TABLE 6.4.   Samples of Time-Management Applications   178

TABLE 7.1.   Basic Roles and Responsibilities of Students,   194
Disability Service Providers, and Instructors

TABLE 7.2.   A List of Potential Team Members for Students to Consider   199

TABLE 7.3.   Self-Advocacy Communication Strategies for College Students   207
with Executive Function Problems

Introduction

Several years ago, my research was focused on understanding the executive function and self-regulation problems of adults with traumatic brain injury (TBI). My long-term goal was to figure out therapeutic ways to help adults self-assess and self-manage their own thinking and behavior. As a speech–language pathologist, I knew that poor self-regulation contributes significantly to why clients do not follow through with the strategies that they have learned and are willing to use. Then one day I met a college student on campus who had sustained a TBI. He was managing to get through most of his classes, but he was navigating college alone, without any academic support on campus besides what he received through disability services. We met a few times and, as I listened to his story, I realized that I had something to offer him, and that those years of researching executive functions, metacognition, and self-regulation could turn into something tangibly useful for students like him.

This book is the result of a good deal of thinking about, discussing, and researching executive function problems and, most important, coaching students with brain injury who have these problems. It integrates the scientific *and* the clinical evidence from many disciplines, including education; disabilities studies; educational, cognitive, developmental, and counseling psychology; neuropsychology; cognitive rehabilitation; and speech–language pathology. As such, it is a book that explains a dynamic coaching approach that three other coaches (Miriam Krause, PhD, CCC-SLP; Katy H. O'Brien, PhD, CCC-SLP; and Sarah Schellinger, PhD, CCC-SLP) and I developed over a 6-year period.

But why have you selected a book about coaching college students with executive function problems? Maybe it is because you have noticed that many college

1

students need help with those skills that are considered "executive functions"? Are you a disability specialist on a college campus, a rehabilitation professional, an educator, or a vocational rehabilitation counselor who has observed how challenging college can be for students with executive function problems? If so, this book will help professionals, like you, who are interested in integrating coaching into their practice with this group of college students.

Maybe you are in search of an intervention approach that could result in your clients or students figuring out their own strategies to reach their goals, including creating realistic goals, making doable plans, and using strategies that are based on what they know about their own strengths and weaknesses. While we know that students with brain injury have executive function problems and that these students are growing in numbers on college campuses, we also know that college students with attention-deficit/hyperactivity disorder (ADHD) and learning disabilities (LD) have executive function problems too. In fact, these are the two largest groups of students with disabilities on college campuses today. So, this book can also be used by the professional who works with students with ADHD, LD, and other groups of college students with executive function problems. Even though there are some distinct differences between these students and those with acquired brain injury, the process of coaching students to self-regulate is the same. That is, through collaborative partnerships with students, goals and strategies are individualized; but the *way* in which the coach interacts with, guides, and partners with students is the same, regardless of the student population. This kind of coaching is dynamic; it is a way of instructing that allows for change. After all, that's what college students do best.

Those of us who work in rehabilitation and in postsecondary education are acutely aware of shrinking funds for traditional therapy and tutoring. With the rising cost of healthcare, most insurance companies have limited the number of therapy sessions for which they are willing to pay. Strapped with the high cost of education, most campus tutoring and disability service centers have experienced financial cutbacks even in the face of increasing numbers of students with disabilities attending college. This situation has forced many of these centers to provide what the federal laws require and little else. Fortunately, the dynamic coaching approach described here is much less intensive than traditional rehabilitation therapy and occurs while students are enrolled in college; as such, the overarching goal of this approach is for students to learn how to "coach" themselves.

Furthermore, there has been a big emphasis on supporting students with disabilities as they transition to college because we know how important it is to provide this support as they make this huge change. However, supporting students *while in college* has been largely ignored. The statistics are fairly grim on retaining college students with disabilities, particularly those with cognitive or intellectual impairments. For this reason an additional purpose of this book is to invite and instruct professionals who have discipline-specific backgrounds to learn how to dynamically coach college students to self-regulate, to self-manage and organize their learning, and to advocate for themselves. To do so, I provide professionals with the theoretic framework, scientific evidence, and practical tools for coaching students in self-regulation, the essential element of executive functions.

This book is organized into two parts: foundational information is provided in Part I, and the elements of dynamic coaching are provided in Part II. The first three chapters are foundational to the rest of the book's content. Chapter 1, "Executive Functions and Self-Regulation," provides readers with descriptions and explanations of executive function and self-regulation problems. The relationships between these two aspects of cognition are highlighted, and readers are exposed to various perspectives and terms used to describe each one. Chapter 2, "College Students with Executive Function Problems," describes the affected student populations, including more traditional learners (e.g., students with ADHD) and students with acquired brain injury, particularly those with TBI and postconcussion syndrome. Chapter 3, "Military Service Members and Veterans in College," is written by Donald L. MacLennan, MS, CCC-SLP, and Leslie Nitta, MA, CCC-SLP, who have years of experience working with veterans, including those going to college. This unique population of college students is growing rapidly, and readers are provided with a description of who these students are, the military culture that they come from, and the academic considerations that must be taken into account when working with them. This chapter also describes the experiences of student veterans with blast-related disabilities and postdeployment syndrome.

Part II consists of five chapters that describe the process of coaching and the tools needed to coach students with executive function problems. Chapter 4, "A Dynamic Coaching Approach," introduces readers to the overarching principles of dynamic coaching, including scientific and clinical evidence for its effectiveness. The phases of dynamic coaching are described, as well as the four tenets on which they are based. The Goal–Strategy–Act–Adjust (GSAA) structure that coaches can use to explicitly instruct students in self-regulation is explained in detail. Some generic forms are introduced here that can help guide coaches and students through the GSAA process. Chapter 5, "Information Gathering and Collaborative Planning," starts by describing the kinds of information a coach needs, how to obtain that information, and where to find it. Since much of this information comes directly from students themselves, the coaching actually starts here, at the information-gathering stage. A big part of this coaching stage is determining students' executive function strengths and weaknesses, identifying strategies that they are already using (which may or may not be effective), finding out students' goals and aspirations, and partnering with students to prioritize these goals and come up with specific plans. Questionnaires and forms are provided throughout this chapter to guide coaches through this initial phase.

Chapter 6, "Coaching Self-Management and Self-Learning: Goals–Strategies–Act–Adjust," coauthored with Katy H. O'Brien, PhD, CCC-SLP, and Chapter 7, "Coaching Self-Advocacy," provide coaches with the needed skills for addressing these three domains that are so critical to the success of college students with executive function problems. The focus in each of these chapters is on the entire self-regulation process, and not just on student goals or the strategies to reach those goals. In Chapter 6 we integrate coaching practices as they apply to studying, learning, time management, planning, and organization because in my own practice these areas were often inseparable. Chapter 7 provides information that coaches need to know about help-seeking behavior in college students with disabilities and about the rights and responsibilities of students and disability service specialists related to reasonable accommodations. Coaches are provided with examples of how to use the GSAA to coach students to self-advocate with disability service providers, instructors, and friends.

Chapter 8, "Coaching toward Independence," concludes the book, with some final suggestions for fostering self-coaching, as students become more independent self-regulators, particularly when they seem to be "stuck." Finally, readers are asked to consider how they will integrate dynamic coaching into their current clinical or education practice by exploring the perceived or real barriers and identifying potential solutions.

PART I
FOUNDATIONS

CHAPTER 1

Executive Functions and Self-Regulation

In this first chapter I introduce readers to executive functions and explain the integral role that self-regulation plays. The relationships between executive function and self-regulation are critically important to understand, considering the dynamic and fluid nature of these skills in the academic, work, and social life of college students. The various aspects of both of these subtypes of cognition not only help us understand the deficits in each, but also inform us about how college students can be coached in order to optimize their own academic and social success. The purpose of this chapter is to provide readers with this foundational knowledge on which the dynamic coaching approach is based. Therefore, the objectives of this chapter are:

- To provide readers with an understanding of what executive functions are and what impairments of executive functions look like in college students.

- To provide readers with an understanding of self-regulation as fluid and ongoing cognitive operations that are central to executive functions.

- To describe for readers the relationships between the beliefs one has about oneself (called self-awareness or self-efficacy) as compared to the ongoing and intentional processes of self-monitoring, self-control, implementing strategies and plans, and comparing and adjusting.

- To describe for readers the importance of self-regulation for college students and why it is the focus of our coaching approach.

WHAT ARE EXECUTIVE FUNCTIONS?

There are several acceptable definitions of executive functions that have emerged from various fields, including neuropsychology and educational, developmental, and cognitive psychology. But to understand what executive functions are and what they do, we must first understand that executive functions exist within a broader framework of cognition. The most common framework is one posited by Stuss and Benson in 1986, over 30 years ago. Based on the work of Luria (1973, 1980) in the mid-20th century, the components of cognition are viewed as a hierarchy that includes both basic and higher-level thinking skills. In this representation, a "sense of self" is the highest level of cognition—this is how we perceive ourselves and is typically operationalized as "self-awareness." More basic cognitive, language, and motor processes are represented at the bottom of the hierarchy. These include attention, alertness, visuospatial skills, memory, language, perception, emotional processes, and motor skills. Table 1.1 provides brief definitions of each of these processes and how impairments in each might appear in the behavior of a college student. For example, a student with impaired memory ability to store information is capable of understanding a lecture, but will struggle to retain the information at a later time. While most students are challenged to learn all that is required of them, students with memory impairment are particularly disadvantaged. A student who has difficulty paying attention may appear to have difficulty remembering material presented in class; thus, while it may look like a memory impairment, the underlying problem is inattention, making it difficult to get information into one's memory for later recall.

Thus, cognitive, sensory, language, and motor impairments result in a wide variety of disabilities. The practical effects of these disabilities on students' academic and social experiences are listed in Table 1.1. Note that these disabilities are examples only; this is not an all-inclusive list of disabilities that result from these impairments.

What can college students do about these disabilities? Besides getting reasonable accommodations for their disabilities, which can help compensate for them (see Chapter 7), students must enlist the help of their own executive functions. Students with memory impairment can recruit the various executive functions (in the middle of the hierarchy) that help them to plan ahead and take good notes, to record lectures, and to use effective study and test-taking strategies. Disabilities tend to create obstacles and barriers, whereas executive functions are the tools that allow us to overcome these obstacles (Ylvisaker, 1998).

In the Stuss and Benson (1986) model, executive functions moderate the ability to compensate for disabilities created by more basic impairments, be they motor, cognitive, language, or emotional, for example. To do this, they operate in the middle, between the sense of self or self-awareness and basic processes. The

TABLE 1.1. Cognitive, Language, Physical, and Sensory Processes and How Impairments in These Domains May Manifest in Students' Ability to Succeed Academically and Socially in College

Cognitive process	Students with these impairments may . . .
Attention: Focusing on a specified activity, behavior, or task. Levels from basic to complex include focused, sustained, alternating, and divided.	• Be distractible during class, while studying, or during conversation. • Talk out of turn. • Have a low tolerance for frustration. • Not follow through on assignments or personal commitments.
Visuospatial: Understanding and being able to mentally manipulate visual information, such as understanding spatial relationships, discriminating items or features, or recognizing objects.	• Complete reading assignments slowly or with great difficulty. • Fatigue easily when reading. • Struggle to interpret figures or graphs. • Only partially recall graphically displayed information. • Organize notes poorly when taking notes from lectures.
Alertness: Maintaining arousal.	• Fall asleep during class or while studying. • Fluctuate alertness during academic activities, resulting in inconsistent comprehension and recall. • Require frequent rest periods, especially after periods of cognitive effort (like class or exams). • Not be able to tolerate infrequent and lengthy classes, such as 3-hour classes that meet once a week. • Require more time to complete work.
Memory: Gathering information so that it can be stored and then recalled at a later time.	• Have difficulty recalling facts and new information for tests. • Forget what is read. • Be unable to connect information and draw inferences when reading. • Not know when assignments are due. • Not remember classmates' names. • Get their schedule confused, so that they arrive at the wrong class on the wrong day or at the wrong location. • Rely on poor memory strategies, such as repetition, when studying. • Complete assignments, but forget to turn them in or misplace them. • Confuse information from one class with information they are learning in another class. • Alienate friends by forgetting to go to social engagements.
Autonomic/emotional: Internal mood or feelings, including automatic responses.	• Have test anxiety. • Avoid groups, make few personal connections with classmates or professors. • Experience cognitive "side effects" from anxiety or depression, such as increased difficulty recalling information. • Allow academic failures to easily undermine their self-efficacy as a student. • Have low resiliency for challenging situations. • Display negative coping behaviors, such as avoidance, eating too much or too little, drinking alcohol or caffeine excessively.

(continued)

TABLE 1.1. *(continued)*

Cognitive process	Students with these impairments may . . .
	• Compulsively check papers or assignments for errors, even if this extra checking results in the assignment being turned in late. • Have difficulty balancing academic and social life.
Sensory/perceptual: General sensory input such as the sensation of touch or proprioception (knowing where the body is in space). Specific sensory input such as vision and hearing.	• Struggle to understand speech because of background noise, particularly during group work. • Avoid conversations with peers if unable to hear clearly. • Not be able to see slides or notes on a whiteboard. • Have difficulty reading textbooks. • Have difficulty manipulating writing materials. • Require preferred seating in classes. • Not enjoy many typical college experiences because of sensory overload (e.g., avoid football games, noisy parties, or restaurants).
Language: Expressive language includes thinking of words, sequencing the sounds in the words, then organizing them into grammatically correct sentences; speaking at an appropriate rate and with intonation consistent for the intended meaning. Receptive language includes comprehending speech and decoding meaning—both explicit and implicit—based on factors such as emphasis, facial or body expressions, and intonation. Also being able to read and write fluently.	• Be slow to respond to questions. • Become frustrated by group interactions that require listening and responding to multiple speakers. • Learn new vocabulary slowly. • Ramble or use nonspecific speech such as "stuff" or "things" when searching for a word. • Struggle to understand lectures, but be hesitant to ask clarification questions. • Need to sit at the front of the class to hear the instructor clearly and use visual input to maximize listening comprehension. • Use a note taker or swap notes with classmates after class so that they do not have to listen, comprehend, and write simultaneously. • Have difficulty understanding implicit information when reading texts. • Focus on explicit information in texts while missing implicit information. • Require support to write and edit lengthy papers. • Make frequent grammatical and spelling errors when writing.
Motor: Planning and executing motor movements, involving the limbs, hands, face, or tongue.	• Be slow to take notes in class. • Need extra time to write papers or emails on a computer because typing is slower than their stream of thought. • Struggle to speak intelligibly with peers in informal settings or during more formal activities, like giving class presentations. • Require extra time to travel between classes or to find a seat in class. • Have to select a seat in class based on motoric needs rather than cognitive needs (e.g., sitting at the back to allow room for a wheelchair, rather than sitting at the front where they could hear more clearly).

terminology used to refer to skills encapsulated by executive functions varies, but includes such abilities as anticipating, goal setting, planning, and monitoring. Executive functions are the controllers of the basic skills, and as such direct, assess, and make decisions about what to attend to, how to subtly respond to a sensitive question, which goals are more important than others, how to initiate use of strategies, how to compare results with goals, and so on. However, executive functions are also dependent on the more basic processes. For example, a typical student needs to be able to maintain attention to read a text, but executive functions direct attention toward the text while also working to make decisions about what pieces of information might be most important. In contrast, if a student has a severe memory impairment for which he is unable to retain new information, his ability to set goals and make strategic decisions will suffer, since these kinds of decisions depend to an extent on an accurate recall of what has happened recently. This also means that students may manifest difficulty at the basic systems level and at the executive functions middle level. These students have *dual disabilities*: an impairment of basic cognitive processes and an impairment of executive functions, the very processes that help them figure out how to compensate or maneuver around their disability.

Neuropsychology and rehabilitation disciplines (e.g., speech–language pathology and occupational therapy) have emphasized the integrative nature of executive functions that allows one to "determine goal-directed and purposeful behavior in everyday life." These processes include inhibition, working memory, shifting thoughts and/or actions, generating goals, planning, reasoning, self-control, and "monitoring and adaptive behavior to fit a particular task or context" (Cicerone et al., 2000, p. 1605).

Regardless of how executive functions are defined, there is no doubt that many of these processes are interrelated. An analysis of a wide range of executive function tasks by young and old adults in 2000 revealed that these functions are fundamentally related to three categories of behavior: shifting, updating and monitoring information, and inhibiting (Miyake, Friedman, Emerson, Witzki, & Howerter, 2000). More recently, Hofmann, Schmeichel, and Baddeley (2012) reviewed the factors included in various models of executive functions and concluded that three common features account for the variability across models:

1. *Working memory,* defined as the ability to hold, manipulate, and update information internally.

2. *Inhibition,* defined as the ability to withhold or to disengage from behaving or thinking based on impulses or routines.

3. *Mental set shifting,* defined as the ability to switch back and forth from one kind of behavior or thought pattern to another.

Others have found that executive functions can be grouped into two broad categories: behavioral regulation and metacognition both in children (Gioia, Isquith, Guy, & Kenworthy, 2002) and in adults (Roth, Lance, Isquith, Fischer, & Giancola, 2013). Using a questionnaire called the Behavior Rating Inventory of Executive Function (BRIEF), researchers found that all of the items were interrelated to each other in one of two ways: *regulating behavior* and *regulating thinking (metacognition)*.

For the purposes of this book, the executive functions and examples of what impairments may look like in the behavior of college students are listed in Table 1.2. This list comes from our knowledge of the research and are commonly identified as contributing to daily life experiences in young adults and in our work with college students with executive function problems. For example, a student who has memory impairment with poor cognitive self-regulation may underestimate the amount of time and effort it will take to study for an exam and will fare worse than a student with memory impairment with strong cognitive self-regulation who plans ahead, adjusts her study schedule, and knows that more effort will be needed. Thus, students with cognitive, motor, sensory, language, and emotional disabilities, who nevertheless have the capability to succeed in college, need strong executive function skills so that they can anticipate problems and create solutions around the barriers created by their disability. As pointed out earlier, students who have executive function problems in addition to their other disabilities have dual disabilities. The manifestations of executive function problems that are listed in Table 1.2 are examples of the kinds of problems college students may have.

Why are there so many different lists of executive functions? There are three primary reasons for this. First and foremost, the definitions reflect the efforts of researchers from various disciplines to modify the original framework of Luria (1980) and Stuss and Benson (1986) based on advances in science and education. Although the lists have been modified, the notion that executive functions oversee more basic systems to manage daily problems, while as the same time receive input from these same systems, has been a challenging concept to test. On the other end of the hierarchy, the integration and influence of one's sense of self or self-awareness has face validity but is hard to prove. We are indeed closer to understanding the contributions to executive functions made by more basic cognitive processes on the one end, and self-awareness on the other end, given that the scientific and educational communities are more accepting (and even embracing) of using a mix of test results, interviews, and questionnaires to find out what individuals think about their thinking and why.

Second, executive functions are developmental by nature, and the labels given to the executive functions seem to change across the lifespan. Emerging executive functions in children are solidified in early adulthood. Neurobiologically, the structural architecture of cortical gray matter and the connections in white matter reach maturation in the frontal lobes of the brain in young adults (Barnea-Goraly

TABLE 1.2. Executive Functions and How Impairments in These Domains May Be Manifest in Students' Abilities in College

Executive functions	Students may . . .
Attention control: Deciding what to pay attention to, what to ignore, how long to attend, and when to switch attention.	• Get too focused on one part of an assignment. • Be easily distracted in class, during exams, and while studying. • Become distracted when completing long assignments. • Not recall or learn material.
Memory control: Holding information in one's mind in order to manipulate it; retrieving details when needed; or remembering to do something at a later time (i.e., prospective memory).	• Not be able to follow a threaded discussion or lengthy instructions or texts. • Have trouble multitasking (e.g., listening and taking notes). • Make decisions based on limited information. • Forget to do assignments and to plan. • Forget important details. • Miss punch lines or story conclusions because they do not recall previous important information. • Have difficulty weighing options.
Initiation: Acting and following through in response to a reminder or recollection.	• Appear lazy or unmotivated. • Have trouble starting or restarting assignments. • Not seek for help from others. • Appear to procrastinate.
Inhibition and impulse control: Withholding the urge to say or do something that does not fit the circumstance or seems out of place.	• Make snap decisions, jump to conclusions. • Complete assignments quickly without checking them. • Say what comes to mind without considering the situation. • Respond quickly, "in the moment" instead of "wait and see."
Problem identification and goal setting: Knowing when there is a problem, deciding on goals, and creating smaller goals/tasks in order to meet the goal.	• Not recognize when a problem exists. • Identify general problems (e.g., having trouble with writing), but cannot identify why or the steps to solve it. • Generate lots of goals, but cannot sequence them into logical steps, especially for large assignments. • Not be able to break down a goal into the smaller steps needed to achieve it.
Flexibility in thinking and behavior: Being able to switch one's former or routine viewpoint, behavior, and way of thinking.	• May not perceive that a different way of thinking or behaving could help remedy a problem situation. • Get stuck in a routine, especially when studying and socializing. • Start but not be able to maintain a new routine. • Appear self-centered. • Have difficulty returning to a routine if it is interrupted.
Emotion self-regulation: Managing and bouncing back from everyday ups and downs without overreacting.	• React emotionally in ways that are out of proportion to the situation. • Get upset or overly discouraged when given feedback. • Have fluctuating emotions or "mood swings" over a short period of time. • Get easily irritated if someone disagrees with them.
Cognitive self-regulation: Monitoring the need for strategies; selecting and implementing strategies.	• Underestimate the need to study and to use strategies for learning. • Underestimate the amount of time and effort it takes to complete assignments and to study for exams. • Not adjust or change study strategies even when current ones are ineffective. • Know about a number of study strategies that could be useful, but do not use them.

et al., 2005). And even though the brain changes throughout adulthood through what we now understand as neuroplasticity, the underlying structural foundation is fairly complete by the mid-20s (Lebel & Beaulieu, 2011). The demands of the environment (at school, work, and play) change: Children who were dependent on their family to assist them in executive functioning are suddenly expected to take over these executive functions as they exert their independence, rely more on peer feedback, and navigate more challenging contexts. We also know that the experiences we have also change how our brain will respond at a future point in time. Conversely, as one becomes an older adult, some aspects of cognition decline (Salthouse, Atkinson, & Berish, 2003). So definitions of executive functions may also reflect the age group from which that definition was derived.

Third, executive functions are affected by differences in or disorders of neurobiology. Individuals with neurodevelopmental disorders, such as ADHD, have certain kinds of executive function challenges that are different from those individuals who have intellectual disabilities. Individuals with acquired brain injury, including TBI, stroke, tumors, encephalitis, or progressive neurological diseases (e.g., multiple sclerosis), have unique executive function deficits based on the age of the individuals when the injury occurred, the type and severity of the injury, the location of the injury in the brain, and the recovery pattern or progression of the disease. Thus, definitions of executive functions reflect the population sample on which the research was based.

As we noted previously, we know that these processes work in concert to self-assess, make strategy decisions, distribute attention, initiate action, block out distractions, shift attention, exert effort, create goals, follow through with an action plan, make adjustments in response to feedback (self or external), and hold information in working memory to allow for reasoning and decision making—all done with seemingly little effort so as to maximize performance in a given activity. There is wide agreement that these are critically important ways of thinking and behaving that can have positive or negative effects on how we function in the world. This is especially true for the college student who has a disability. For the purposes of this book, executive function domains are described in Table 1.2, including examples of possible student behaviors associated with difficulties in each of these domains.

However, executive functions are not involved in all kinds of behavior. Automatic behaviors and routines, wherein one does not consider or think about what should be done, are based on long-term memory that has been solidified through years of repeating the same behavior or as a conditioned response (Squire, 1992). These responses and behaviors are fast, seemingly automatic, and under little cognitive or conscious control. Examples of these kinds of behaviors include brushing your teeth as a part of your morning routine, driving a car, or even having memories about a past Thanksgiving dinner as soon as you smell the aroma of the turkey in the oven. College students can have many routines in place, such as taking notes during class, drilling with flashcards to study, or packing books and computers for class each morning. Maladaptive routines can also be established, such as cramming before exams or writing papers the night before rather than using executive functions to plan and study over a more appropriate period of time. College students with or without disabilities may rely on old routines that worked well for them in high school, but have become ineffective when met with the demands of college. Students without executive function disabilities can figure out what is or is not working and make adjustments, whereas students with executive function problems lack the skills to figure this out on their own.

WHAT IS SELF-REGULATION AND HOW IS IT RELATED TO EXECUTIVE FUNCTIONS?

Self-regulation is the ability to assess one's own (hence the "self") cognitive and emotional states and to make decisions about what to do in light of that assessment. Self-regulation is a group of cognitive considerations and are the "meta" manipulations that allow us to monitor and control our own emotions, thoughts, and actions. Rather than viewing self-regulation as one of many executive functions, as Cicerone and colleagues (2000) described above, we view self-regulation as integrally related to the executive function processes required to carry out everything from simple to complex intentional actions. Self-regulation occurs within a context and is a limited resource, wherein students must make both quick learning decisions and slow, more planful ones. Readers who wish to explore this aspect of self-regulation further are referred to a special issue of *Metacognition Learning* that is dedicated to the complexities of self-regulated learning (Ben-Eliyahu & Bernacki, 2015).

Self-regulation is sometimes used synonymously with *metacognition,* or thinking about your thinking when referring to cognition, and *metamemory,* or thinking about your memory and learning. Sometimes self-regulation is interpreted as only including "self-control," or withholding or not engaging in a routinized or impulsive behavior, like overeating, or not blurting out what we really think. Self-regulation is viewed by cognitive, developmental, and educational psychologists as including both self-monitoring and self-control.

Flavell (1979) was a developmental psychologist who conceptualized self-regulation as having two parts. He described ongoing "metacognitive experiences" as those that occur during our daily lives at school, home, and work and in the community during activities in which we engage. These experiences can be divided into two parts: self-monitoring, or self-assessment, and self-control, or the ability to decide to act in a particular way. In the Stuss and Benson (1986) framework, these processes are implicitly inherent in the executive functions in the middle of their model, but with an emphasis on self-monitoring and self-control. The second part of Flavell's conceptualization is metacognitive or autobiographical "beliefs." These are the stored memories of those daily experiences that become integrated into what we believe about ourselves. These include ideas about what we are good at and not good at doing and what strategies have been successful or not. Neuropsychologists might call this the "sense of self" and operationalize it as "self-awareness." Flavell also stressed the interaction between these two; that metacognitive experiences serve to update our metacognitive beliefs or sense of self.

Since then, psychologists, educators, and rehabilitation professionals have considered how ongoing self-regulation interacts with one's goals and one's motivation to figure out a problem or engage in complex activities (Carver & Scheier, 2001; Evans, Kirby, & Fabrigar, 2003). Carver and Scheier (1991) summarized two connotations of self-regulation that fit here: one is "the sense of self-corrective adjustments being made as the person [actively] interacts with the world," and the other is a sense of purpose as in goal-directed behavior (p. 168). Kennedy and Coelho (2005) used these conceptualizations of self-regulation to describe its underlying processes and the potential points of breakdown involved in intentional, complex activities for individuals with executive function problems from an acquired brain injury (e.g., TBI, stroke). Seen here as a cycle or sequence of behaviors, this is the self-regulation model used throughout this book. Figure 1.1 is a modification of the 2005 conceptualization. It shows the ongoing relationships between self-monitoring, self-control, taking action, comparing performance with the goal, and making adjustments. For a discussion of theories that have informed our approach,

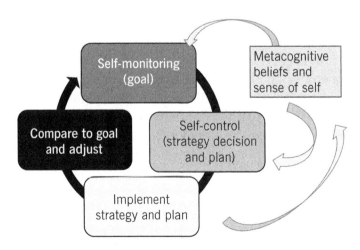

FIGURE 1.1. Model of self-regulation. Based on Kennedy and Coelho (2005).

readers are also referred to Hart and Evans (2006). Each part of this model is operationalized in the following manner:

- Self-monitoring, or self-assessing, is done by considering or predicting how one will do based on past experiences and the demands of the task. If one thinks that he or she will not perform as well as wanted, then a goal is established. If one thinks that he or she will perform well, then there is no reason for a goal. Creating a goal actually triggers the sequence of thinking "events" or steps in the rest of the sequence (e.g., Locke & Latham, 2002).
- Self-control, or making strategy decisions, is linked to self-monitoring. When one self-assesses the need for a goal, then one needs to make a strategic decision (i.e., use the same strategy as used before, or use a different strategy).
- Acting, or implementing the strategy plan.
- Comparing the results with the goal occurs when getting feedback. Feedback can be self-generated (using self-monitoring) or externally generated (e.g., instructor or employer feedback). Regardless of the type of feedback, willingness to self-monitor is again a key component in this step. If the goal was reached, then there is no need to adjust the goal or the strategy. However, if the goal was not reached, then either the goal or the strategy needs adjustment (i.e., change the goal *or* select and implement a different strategy).

Take, as an example, a common metacognitive experience of the college student who is studying. She assesses the situation (self-monitors) and realizes that she is going to need to put forth effort into studying for an upcoming exam, so she decides to use a strategy (self-control) (e.g., reviewing class notes) and selects one that has worked well for her in the past. However, when the exam grade is lower than she expected (compares outcome with her goal), she decides that she will need to use a different strategy (self-control) the next time if she wants to achieve her goal. The discrepancy between her goal and her performance, that is, a lower grade than expected, forces her to consider a different study approach if her goal remains the same. However, she could also reduce her performance expectations for the next exam and stick with the same study strategy. In both of these scenarios, she has made adjustments and thereby reduced the discrepancy between her goal and her performance (Carver & Scheier, 1991).

In the model shown in Figure 1.1, metacognitive beliefs, or self-awareness, have both influenced the metacognitive experiences and have also been affected by them. How might this work? The student in the above example viewed herself as academically strong (metacognitive beliefs) and as one who could rely on a simple strategy like reviewing class notes. This is what had worked well in the past, and she saw no reason to change that strategy now. In this way, her sense of self and past experiences influenced her choice of strategies. However, when the results fell short of what she expected, she could either adjust the goal (e.g., I'm fine with getting a lower grade) or she could select a different strategy, one that would improve the chances of her getting a more acceptable grade. If her perception of herself (also called self-efficacy) is strong, meaning she believes she has the capability of getting a better grade, then she is likely to choose a different study strategy, perhaps one that she has used before when material is difficult, such as creating note cards and using them to self-quiz. To prepare for the next exam, she uses note cards and her exam grade improves. These experiences will not likely change her sense of self as a strong student, but it may show her that in some situations where the demands are greater, she simply has to use a different strategy, one that takes more time and effort. And while underlying her belief that she is a strong student may not change, this experience has enriched and deepened her awareness that she *is capable of figuring this out and being successful.*

Self-efficacy, or self-determination, is a critical aspect of self-awareness and is used to operationalize the belief that "I will be successful" or "I will figure this out." The broader-based construct of "self-determination," however, captures both the ongoing self-assessment and adjustment of self-regulation as well as the self-efficacy or beliefs that one holds about oneself. Self-determination is

> a combination of skills, knowledge and beliefs that enable a person to engage in goal-directed, self-regulated, autonomous behavior. An understanding of one's strengths and limitations together with a belief in oneself as capable and effective are essential to self-determination. When acting on the basis of these skills and attitudes, individuals have better ability to take control of their lives and assume the role of successful adults. (Field, Martin, Miller, Ward, & Wehmeyer, 1998, p. 115)

Indeed, individuals with strong self-determination are more likely to put more effort into and be more persistent in accomplishing their goals than those with low self-determination (Bandura, 1997). Yet, students also need to be able to create doable goals and have the knowledge, plans, and skills to accomplish their goals (Schunk, 1991).

Self-regulating emotions are an important factor that can have positive or negative consequences for the ability to engage in cognitive self-regulation, which has been the center of our discussion so far. Emotion regulation is the ability to self-monitor and self-control one's emotional states. When an emotion such as anxiety occurs, it can have a negative effect on an individual's self-control. Wyble, Sharma, and Bowman (2008) described a neural network of emotional self-regulation that can interfere with the ability to make self-control decisions in the cognitive domains. They showed that negative emotional interference during a taxing cognitive-control task (i.e., the Stroop task) can slow down, suppress, or even withdraw their attention from the challenging task. In college, students may get a lot of negative feedback if they are struggling academically or socially. This negativity can then result in the likelihood that they will disengage or withdraw from those situations or activities, explained by Wyble and colleagues as a protective or defense mechanism. Thus, having the support of a coach and a team of individuals to whom these students can turn is even more important for these students than for students who are doing well in college and receive positive feedback. Furthermore, preventing negative experiences from occurring in the first place can be a key element of supporting college students with executive function problems.

Why Emphasize Self-Regulation?

Self-regulation is the ability to assess, select, act, adapt, and understand how "the self" has input into these processes. Self-regulation is a set of processes that are at the core of executive functions. Consider the current college and work environments. The successful student or employee is one who follows the rules but can quickly assess, look for options, and adapt on demand. This fluid form of intelligence actually predicts learning in both settings. A meta-analysis conducted by Sitzman and Ely (2011) found that four aspects of self-regulation had the strongest effect or impact on learning and work:

1. Identifying and setting attainable goals.
2. Being persistent in the steps taken toward those goals.
3. Appropriating and maintaining good effort or motivation.
4. Having the self-efficacy that they have the knowledge and skills to be successful.

In this sense, self-regulation "reflects goal-oriented behavior and includes a multitude of processes operating in concert . . . within a learning context" (Sitzman & Ely, 2011, p. 421). Here, the context is college.

In general, self-regulation in high school and college students appears to be related to general academic success and adjustment. Those students with self-regulation abilities are more likely to graduate and have higher GPAs compared to students without these kinds of abilities (Getzel & Thoma, 2008; Kitsanta, Winsler, & Huie, 2008). In a review of what contributes to university students' GPA, Richardson, Abraham, and Bond (2012) found that self-efficacy predicted GPA the best, followed by students' high school GPA. Additionally, all three aspects of self-regulation (self-efficacy, having goals, and effort regulation) positively correlated with GPA.

Furthermore, several studies point out the relationship between self-regulation and academic stress in older high school students and in college students. For example, Kadzikowska-Wrzosek (2012) found that of 18- to 19-year-olds who experienced test-taking stress but had used self-regulation strategies had fewer mental health problems when compared to stressed students who did not use self-regulation skills. Others have found that in the first year of college, students who improved in their self-regulation abilities (constructive thinking or problem solving, emotion regulation, and sense of mastery) were better adjusted psychologically at the end of the first year compared to students who did not improve in self-regulation (Park, Edmundson, & Lee, 2011).

Unfortunately, individuals appear to have a limited capacity for self-regulation. Over 600 studies in the social and behavior sciences have shown that self-control, the ability to suppress thoughts or behaviors in favor of those that are needed to meet a goal, can be depleted. In other words, we have a set amount of self-regulation resources, and when we run out, we are less likely to be able to inhibit or use self-control (Muraven & Baumeister, 2000). For college students, the need for self-control can be very demanding. Students have to exert discipline to study, to get to class on time, to meet deadlines, to engage in healthy living behaviors, to say no, at times, to friends, and so forth. However, stress, which is a part of college life, impairs or depletes self-control. Students who experience high levels of exam stress, for example, tend to smoke more (West & Lennox, 1992) and exercise less (Steptoe, Wardle, Pollard, Canaan, & Davies, 1996) before exams. These two behaviors require self-control: for the latter, students were unable to exert self-control over smoking, and for the former, students did not exert self-control by continuing to exercise. Oaten and Cheng (2005) found that students who were stressed during exams were more likely to engage in more unhealthy eating, smoking, and drinking of caffeine, and had less emotional control, a lack of follow-through to commitments, and poor study habits, for example. When professionals working with college students have a better understanding of detrimental effects that stress has on self-regulation, they can help students to develop a stress management plan to prevent self-regulation fatigue during critical times in the semester.

For college students without disabilities, self-regulation usually predicts academic success. For individuals with disabilities, having strong executive functions, specifically self-regulation skills, is even more critical to their success. For students with disabilities such as hearing, visual, and mobility impairments, those who have strong executive function abilities can compensate for and work around their disabilities and overcome many of the barriers to learning, socializing, and working. However, students *with executive function disabilities* lack the very self-regulation skills that would improve the likelihood of their success; they lack these critical *ways of thinking and problem solving*. Highlighting the need to emphasize these self-skills, Ylvisaker (1998) stated, "What you do with what you have is more important than what you have." In other words, for students who have the basic cognitive, language, and memory abilities to learn college-level material, *how they use their strengths and compensate for their weaknesses is more critical to college success than what their strengths and weaknesses are.*

In summary, executive functions are viewed as higher-order cognitive processes that oversee more basic cognitive abilities. And while there are many definitions and lists of executive function skills, self-regulation is a group of processes that are inherent to executive functions. Self-regulation includes both ongoing regulating processes (self-monitoring, self-control, self-acting, and self-comparing/ adjusting) and the sense of oneself, or what one believes about oneself. In complex and intentional activities, self-regulation is necessary in order to create goals, select strategies, plan and sequence the necessary steps, carry out the steps using strategies, evaluate performance using strategies, and make adjustments when necessary. As a part of self-regulation, strong self-efficacy and self-determination are predictors of success not only in college but also at work. The ability to self-regulate is important for all college students, but for those with disabilities, it is critical. However, students with executive function disabilities are at a unique disadvantage since the nature of their disability lies in the very cognitive processes that would allow them to problem-solve, compensate, and adjust to the academic, work, and social demands of college life.

Let us now turn to the groups of college students who are likely to have executive function problems as the result of an acquired condition (e.g., brain injury) or as the result of a developmental condition (e.g., ADHD) in Chapter 2.

College Students
with Executive Function Problems

Now that you have an understanding of executive functions and self-regulation and how these skills may appear in college students, let's describe the types of college students who are likely to have disabilities involving these skills. Many college students may struggle with aspects of executive function, regardless of whether they have an identifiable disability. Few students entering college are truly prepared for the demands that college brings. However, over time, typical students tend to adapt to the college setting, making adjustments to routines to successfully complete academic work and maintain social connections. In fact, when we think of the benefits of a college degree, only some of the benefits are due to the content of the courses. The rest is due to the development of complex, flexible executive function routines that can be used in a variety of work, school, and social settings. This type of executive function development is often referred to as "maturity." Students with executive function problems, though, are not only unprepared for college settings, but they do not have the skills needed to figure out how to meet these academic demands. Therefore, they lack these necessary skills and struggle to make self-adjustments to become the students they would like to be.

The primary objective in this chapter is to describe college students who have executive function problems within the context of all college students with disabilities. The National Center for Education Statistics (NCES; Raue & Lewis, 2011) reported that a total of 3,680 (88% of 4,170) institutions enrolled a total of 707,000 students with disabilities in 2008–2009. Figure 2.1 provides statistics on the percentage of postsecondary institutions that enrolled students by disability category from highest to lowest. With a range of categories from 86% to 41%, it is notable that nearly 50% or more of institutions do not report having any students with TBI,

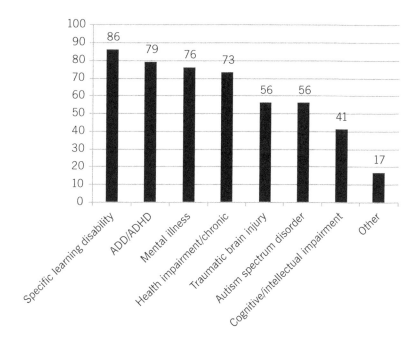

FIGURE 2.1. The percentage of postsecondary institutions with enrolled college students by disability category (Raue & Lewis, 2011).

autism spectrum disorder (ASD), cognitive/intellectual impairment, or "other" kinds of disabilities. What is even more surprising is that not *all* postsecondary institutions report having enrolled students with learning disabilities or ADHD, clearly the largest group of students with disabilities on college campuses!

Figure 2.2 displays the percentages of students by disability category from most to least. Given the lack of reporting of some student disability groups, the figure tells us that the number of students with disabilities is likely an *underrepresentation of the actual number of college students with disabilities.* Registering with disability student services is optional and may be one reason why these numbers are low, given the total population size. Furthermore, certain subgroups of students may be more or less likely to seek support from disability services; these numbers may not reflect the true distribution of any one group of students with disabilities on college campuses. The reasons for not seeking support from disability student services are discussed further in Chapter 7. Kennedy, Krause, and Turkstra (2008) found that nearly 50% of college students with TBI were not familiar with disability student services or had never accessed these services.

Let's consider these groups of students by time of onset of their disability to see how that might impact them. The largest groups of college students with disabilities are those with developmental disabilities: students with ADHD, LD, cognitive/intellectual impairment, and ASD. According to the statistics in Figure 2.2,

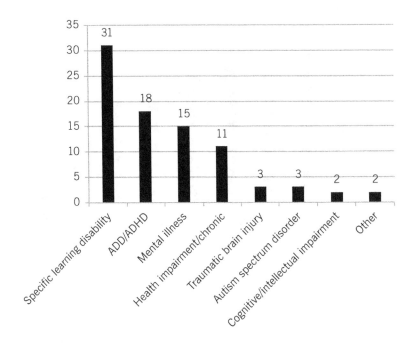

FIGURE 2.2. The percentage of students by disability category at postsecondary institutions (Raue & Lewis, 2011).

this group accounts for 54% of the college students with disabilities. Other groups of students acquire their disability either in late adolescence or early adulthood.

In our experience, considering students with executive function problems in this way reveals some clear differences between these two student groups that impact the kinds of executive function problems they experience in college and how they view their own disability. Students who enter college with developmental disabilities likely had educational support and accommodations throughout elementary, middle, and/or high school, including special education and even transition teams. They have lived with their disability for many years and have a more established sense of self based on their experiences in high school than young adults who have more recently acquired a disability. These students also have more established beliefs about strategies that worked or did not work in the past. They may already view themselves as being a "visual learner," or as someone who learns by doing. As such, they may have strong self-awareness, including self-determination. What they lack is an understanding of how they will navigate college, where the demand for strong executive functions is great and where the amount of support has diminished. "As students transition to postsecondary environments that provide limited external structure and place greater demands on their internal capacity to organize goal-directed behavior, many students with ADHD and LD encounter an intensified need for support services. This new level of challenge often contrasts sharply with students' high school experiences, where parents, teachers, and school programs provided a high degree of external structure" (Parker & Boutelle, 2009, p. 204). Suddenly, it's up to the students themselves to figure everything out as the demands on their ability to self-regulate become taxed. They are faced with new academic and social challenges for which the old strategies and routines may be ineffective, while the amount and type of support they had in high school has virtually disappeared.

For students who have acquired executive function problems in late adolescence, the demands of college are exacerbated by their lack of understanding or awareness of their abilities and disabilities. As noted earlier, if their disability was acquired in elementary or middle school, they may have received the kinds of supports given to individuals with development disabilities, and their sense of self may be similarly established. But students with an acquired disability late in high school or when beginning college have not lived with their "new brain" long enough to understand what they are capable or incapable of doing, even with supports. These students truly do not have the capability of figuring out what the demands of college are, let alone what strategies they could use to meet those demands. The differences between these two groups of students will affect how they cope with these changes, the way in which we coach them in college, and how much coaching support they need to be successful.

Regardless of whether students acquired the disability as older adolescents or were born with a disability, it is important to remember that most of these students have dual disabilities. In other words, they may have more basic learning, language, cognitive, sensory (e.g., vision, hearing), and physical impairments, but they also have difficulty assessing their learning abilities and using their executive functions to adjust their learning strategies to the demands of the task. Looking back at Tables 1.1 and 1.2, these individuals have deficits in both cognitive processes as well as in the executive functions that control those processes. The impairments manifested in daily college activities look like many of the examples included in these tables, but intervention efforts need to address both aspects of the dual impairments in order to be effective. Let's examine each of the student groups affected by such dual disabilities more closely. First we discuss students with developmental disabilities and their executive function problems, followed by a discussion of students with acquired brain injury and their executive function problems.

COLLEGE STUDENTS WITH DEVELOPMENTAL DISABILITIES AND EXECUTIVE FUNCTION PROBLEMS

Students with LD and ADHD are the largest groups of college students with disabilities who are likely to have executive function problems. By definition, an individual with a specific LD is one who has an impairment discrepancy between their overall intelligence, an area of academic achievement, and an area of cognitive processing (Association on Higher Education and Disability [AHEAD], 2000). Individuals with LD may or may not have executive function problems. On the contrary, it has long been held that individuals with ADHD/attention-deficit disorder (ADD) have self-regulation disorders that impact their ability to control their behavior and their emotions as a result of underlying executive function problems (e.g., Barkley, 1997). For example, Wallace, Winsler, and NeSmith (1999) found that self-confidence (self-efficacy), fulfilling student responsibilities that require executive functions (e.g., meeting deadlines, following assignment instructions), and age were the best predictors of GPA in college students with ADHD.

ADHD is present across the lifespan and is characterized as developmental inattention and/or hyperactivity–impulsivity (American Psychiatric Association, 2000). DuPaul, Weyandt, O'Dell, and Varejao (2009) reviewed the prevalence and incidence of ADHD in college students and concluded that between 2 and 8% has ADHD, and that hyperactivity–impulsivity disorders are the most common (DuPaul et al., 2001; Lee, Oakland, Jackson, & Glutting, 2008). If this is true, then there are thousands of students with ADHD and ADD who do not receive support when in college.

For individuals with ADHD/ADD, executive function problems are now considered *the* underlying primary deficit. Willcutt, Doyle, Nigg, Faraone, and Pennington (2005) conducted a meta-analysis of 83 studies that administered common tests of executive function to individuals with ADHD. Across included studies, there were 3,734 individuals with ADHD and 2,969 individuals with no identifiable disability. Individuals with ADHD performed more *poorly on all tests of executive function problems, but impairments of inhibition, vigilance (maintaining attention), working memory, and planning were the most consistent areas of executive function problems.* Not too surprising was the finding of variability; that not all individuals with ADHD had the same kinds of executive function problems. The researchers concluded that

> EF [executive function] weaknesses are significantly associated with ADHD, but they do not support the hypothesis that EF deficits are the single, necessary, and sufficient cause of ADHD in all individuals with the disorder. Instead, EF difficulties appear to be one of several important weaknesses that comprise the overall neuropsychologic etiology of ADHD. (Willcutt et al., 2005, p. 1342)

These underlying executive function processing impairments, along with other executive function problems, such as difficulty solving problems and poor self-regulation, can interfere with academic and social success in college, and these relationships are now well documented (e.g., Barkley, 1990; Butler, 1995).

What are the challenges that college students with ADHD face? DuPaul and colleagues (2009) provided a brief but thorough summary of the research that documents the academic challenges (and social and psychological challenges) students with ADHD have. Academically, these authors found that overall students with ADHD have lower GPAs, have difficulty completing assignments and exams on time, and report working harder to complete assignments when compared to students without disabilities. Others have found that college students with ADHD report self-learning challenges that include a lack of monitoring their own learning, not knowing which study strategies to use and when to use them, and use of ineffective strategies (e.g., Zwart & Kallemeyn, 2001).

Studies showing that students with ADHD experience social challenges in college are mixed. Some have reported that students have lower self-esteem and adjust less well than their nondisabled peers (Shaw-Zirt, Popali-Lehane, Chaplin, & Bergman, 2005), whereas others have reported that they were as satisfied with their social life as their peers in the first year of college (Rabiner, Anastopoulos, Costello, Hoyle, & Swartzwelder, 2008). Regardless, it is unclear that social issues in college students with ADHD are related to executive function problems alone; it is more likely that social issues result from a combination of factors that include personality type, type of ADHD (inattentive or hyperactive), and the specific kind of executive function problem.

Given the overlap between some of the underlying processing impairments of students with ADHD and LD, are there differences between these groups that could affect a coach's approach? Reaser, Prevatt, Petscher, and Proctor (2007) used the Learning and Study Strategies Inventory—2nd Edition (LASSI; Weinstein & Palmer, 2002) to compare study and learning strategies of students with ADHD to students with LD and students without disabilities. There are 10 subscales from the LASSI's 80 items: attitude, motivation, time management, anxiety, concentration, information processing, selecting main ideas, study aids, self-testing, and test strategies. Students without disabilities scored more positively than the two disability groups on all subscales, with the exception of attitude and study aids. The ADHD group scored lower (i.e., worse) than both the LD and the nondisabled group in time management, concentration, selecting main ideas, and test strategies. "The areas in which the students with ADHD reported poorer performance than both groups include two areas that are classic characteristics of ADHD: poor concentration skills and inability to self-regulate and manage one's time" (Reaser et al., 2000, p. 633). But there were areas in which the ADHD group's scores were similar to the LD group, but lower than the nondisabled group: motivation, anxiety, information processing, and self-testing. Thus, students with LD may also need coaching support that consists of less explicit instruction in self-regulation.

Before discussing students with acquired brain injury, it is important to note that students with intellectual disability and ASD may also exhibit executive function problems. Students with intellectual disabilities can attend college with support from both coaches and specifically designed programs to meet their unique learning needs. The numbers of students with ASD on college campuses are likely to grow in the future given the increasing numbers of students in grade school with this disability, the intervention and structured support that these students need throughout school, and the increasing awareness of their specific learning and social abilities and disabilities. Given the amount and kind of support these students now receive in grade school, it is not surprising that many are indeed capable of being successful in college courses. But when they get to college, where this level of support no longer exists, they are ill prepared to manage their own schedule, meet deadlines, and engage in college life.

COLLEGE STUDENTS WITH ACQUIRED BRAIN INJURY AND EXECUTIVE FUNCTION PROBLEMS

Acquired brain injury (ABI) is neurological damage that occurs any time after birth. There are two broad categories of ABI: traumatic and nontraumatic (e.g., stroke, neurological disease). The Centers for Disease Control and Prevention (CDC) state that "a TBI is caused by a bump, blow or jolt to the head or a penetrating head injury that disrupts the normal function of the brain. . . . The severity of a TBI may range from 'mild,' i.e., a brief change in mental status or consciousness to 'severe,' i.e., an extended period of unconsciousness or amnesia after the injury" (*www.cdc.gov/traumaticbraininjury/basics.html*). By this definition, injury severity ranges from concussion to coma. While there is some confusion among the general public on whether or not a concussion is a brain injury, there is no confusion among health-care professionals. Indeed, a concussion is a TBI, just a very mild one. And while the statistics in Figure 2.2 show that only 2% of college students with disabilities in college have TBIs, we know that these numbers are growing.

- Military service members and veterans from recent wars who sustained TBI, including concussion, are returning to college campuses in record numbers using their post-911/GI bill. Chapter 3 describes this special group of college students. Between 2000 and 2011 the Department of Defense estimated that there were 235,046 service members who sustained a TBI (CDC, National Institutes of Health, Department of Defense, & Department of Veterans Affairs Leadership Panel, 2013)

- Young adults with sports-related concussions from football, soccer, and everyday athletic activities are much more likely to receive medical, athletic, rehabilitation, and academic support as best practices are being developed. The CDC estimates that 1.6 to 3.8 million concussions occur each year in the United States in athletic activities (Langlois, Rutland-Brown, & Wald, 2006).

The statistics on TBI in the United States are staggering: 2.2 million individuals sustain a TBI each year. This number includes individuals with concussions from the emergency room data, most of who are symptom-free within a few weeks. There are estimates that 10–15% of those with concussion have lingering, protracted symptoms reporting headaches, fatigue, or difficulty concentrating, called post-concussive syndrome. While children and young adults are most likely to sustain concussions, recent wars in the past decades have resulted in tens of thousands of military service personnel with TBI, including concussion, making it the signature injury of these wars. Vehicular accidents and falls also remain a major cause of TBI, especially of college-age young adults.

The cognitive and communication impairments that are common after TBI include attention disorders, remembering and learning new information, slow processing, word-finding disorders, and executive function disorders (e.g., Draper & Ponsford, 2008). Because of the diffuse injury to the brain during trauma (i.e., many areas of the brain are injured) as well as the size and position/location of the frontal lobes, executive function problems are ubiquitous with TBI. At 1-year postinjury, there are three general groupings or categories of executive function problems common to this population (Busch, McBride, Curtiss, & Vanderploeg, 2005). First, this population experiences a reduction in the ability not only to self-generate behavior, but also to maintain or switch behavior (or responses). Second, these individuals have difficulty with working memory or holding and manipulating information in order to compare, contrast, and solve problems. And last, these individuals have difficulty inhibiting and reporting information that may be inaccurate. And although these three kinds of executive dysfunction are common after moderate to severe TBI, it is also important to acknowledge that each individual and each injury is unique; these are simply the most common kinds of executive function problems associated with TBI. Thus, given the high prevalence of more basic cognitive impairments (e.g., attention, memory, and learning impairments), coupled with additional executive function impairments, it is clear that college students with TBI have dual disabilities. Educational documents such as the one by Kennedy, Vaccaro, and Hart (2015) describe executive function problems in college students with TBI. Although the target audience is disability service providers on college campuses, these documents can be shared with other professionals who are unfamiliar with the impact that TBI and executive function problems can have on college students (*www.partnership.vcu.edu/TBIresources/downloadables/CollegeStudents_TBI.pdf*).

What happens when students with TBI go to college? Unfortunately, the literature is pretty clear; students with TBI struggle academically and socially. They report having to study more and to use more strategies and expend more effort to get the same or lower grades than before their injury (Hux et al., 2010; Kennedy, Krause, & O'Brien, 2014; Mealings, Douglas, & Olver, 2012; Willmott, Ponsford,

Downing, & Carty, 2014). They also report time management issues and difficulties with keeping organized. Because of these problems, they take reduced courseloads, which in turn results in a longer time to earn a degree and higher tuition costs overall if they graduate (Kennedy et al., 2008). Kennedy and colleagues (2014) found that from 13 statements that described challenges in college, four categories emerged: time management and organization; studying and learning; social aspects; and nervousness or stress.

Socially, students with TBI have fewer friends than they had prior to the injury and report that "others do not understand their problems" (Kennedy et al., 2014). Adolescents with TBI engage in fewer social activities than their peers with other disabilities, and their parents report that they withdraw from social situations, take less initiative, and are more likely to be introverted (Turkstra, Politis, & Forsyth, 2015). Although it is tempting to conclude that these consequences are due solely to their cognitive impairments (e.g., memory, speed of processing, executive function problems), it is also the case that these teens are unable to drive for a period of time after being injured, they do not get invited to participate in social activities, and the additional work/effort to keep up with the courseload means that they have less time for socializing (Turkstra et al., 2015).

What about young adults with mild TBI or concussion? Do individuals with mild TBI or concussion have cognitive impairments, including executive function problems? Most individuals with concussion, such as college athletes, experience some cognitive or physical symptoms immediately after or within a few days of being injured (e.g., Covassin, Stearne, & Elbin, 2008). Fortunately, the majority of individuals with concussion experience a full recovery of their initial symptoms within the first few weeks (e.g., Halstead et al., 2013; McClincy, Lovell, Pardini, Collins, & Spore, 2006). For those who do not recover initially, their lingering symptoms can be physical (fatigue, visual disturbances, headaches, imbalance), cognitive (attention problems, slow processing, memory impairment, executive function problems), and psychosocial (irritability, anxiety, depression, frustration, and anger (*www.cdc.gov/headsup/basics/concussion_symptoms.html*). Figure 2.3 displays the possible interactions among these three domains. For example, sensitivity to bright lights is quite common in those with post-concussion syndrome; bright lighting can trigger headaches that can then last for hours or even days. Affected students can get accommodations to wear sunglasses in brightly lit classrooms, but this takes self-advocacy, which they are not used to doing. Also, students with concussion fatigue suddenly may find themselves on campus without a place to rest if they do not have the necessary executive functions (or the energy) to search out quiet places where they can do this. Unfortunately, students with multiple concussions are more likely to have more symptoms, particularly as related to their memory and learning abilities (Iverson, Gaetz, Lovell, & Collins, 2004).

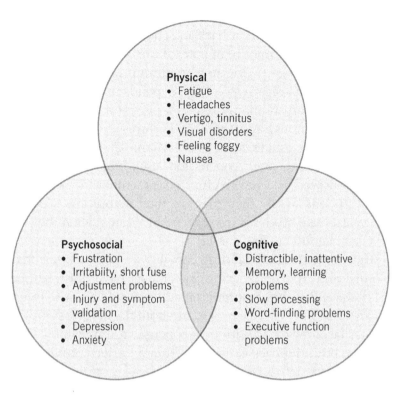

FIGURE 2.3. Three domains of symptoms that interact and overlap after a concussion.

Students with concussion are unprepared to manage these symptoms, in part, because they have not had to before and, in part, because of executive function problems. Many people, even individuals with concussion, are not aware that individuals with concussion can have the same problems with executive functions as individuals with more severe TBI. Knollman-Porter, Constantinidou, and Hutchinson Marron (2014) and others have summarized the symptoms associated with post-concussive syndrome; these include decreases in attentional control, emotion and cognitive self-regulation, working memory, and inhibition. Recently, Donders and Strong (2016) used the Behavior Rating Inventory of Executive Function—Adult Version (BRIEF-A) to explore self-reported executive functions in adults with mild TBI from 1 to 12 months after being injured. They found that three areas of executive functions were impacted: metacognition, behavioral regulation, and emotion regulation. Drake, Gray, Yoder, Pramuka, and Llewellyn (2000) reported that thinking of words quickly, speed in planning and strategizing, and improved memory skills predicted the work status of adults with mild TBI at 3–15 months after their injury. Clearly, executive function problems can be a result of concussion.

There is now consensus that when students with concussion return to school, including college, they should return to school slowly while they manage their symptoms. A slow initial transition back to school may include attending fewer classes initially, reducing the amount of note taking, scheduled periods of rest during the day, and keeping test taking to a minimum until students are symptom free. How quickly students return to college depends on the extent to which their symptoms are being carefully monitored as a part of a concussion management program. Some colleges now have formal procedures and even centers of care for student athletes with concussion, such as the Miami University Concussion Management Program. Students with concussion attending colleges with such programs should be followed by a health clinic staff member that knows how to educate and follow students while they manage their symptoms. Cognitive-activity monitoring logs also help students track their symptoms when they return to college (Master, Gioia, Leddy, & Grady, 2012).

College students with TBI, including concussion, have unique challenges that college personnel and disability service specialists have not traditionally faced. Appendix 2.1 at the end of this chapter is an educational brochure that was created for educators and disability service providers about the unique symptoms and academic challenges faced by those with post-concussive syndrome.

Nontraumatic brain injuries can occur from a variety of neurological events and diseases, including stroke, progressive disease (e.g., multiple sclerosis, Parkinson's disease, and Alzheimer's disease), nonprogressive disease (e.g., encephalitis, meningitis), allergic reactions, and a reduction of oxygen to the brain from trauma or disease elsewhere in the body. In these injuries, executive function problems occur from focal or localized brain damage to specific regions responsible for executive functions, namely the frontal lobes and their white matter connections to the rest of the brain. For example, individuals with left-hemisphere frontal lobe stroke may have language impairment as well as reduced processing speed, initiation, and planning and problem-solving abilities. Individuals with right-hemisphere frontal lobe stroke may have reduced initiation, processing speed, emotion regulation, and reasoning and problem-solving abilities.

In summary, students with executive function problems are attending college in record numbers. Although traditionally most of the students were those with ADHD/ADD and LD, more students with intellectual disabilities and ASD are attending college than ever before. Given the recent attention TBI and concussion has received, many more college students are aware of their deficits and are seeking support while in college. Having learned about the similarities and differences among these student groups, Chapter 3 provides you with an in-depth understanding of college students from military backgrounds who have brain injury and posttraumatic stress disorder (PTSD).

What Disability Service Specialists Should Know about Concussion

Growing numbers of students with concussion are seeking support from college disability service providers. The purpose of this document is to answer some common questions about what to expect when working with college students with concussion. Answers to common questions are provided.

1. **What is a mild TBI (mTBI) or concussion?**
   - CDC task force on mTBI: Any period of observed or self-reported after injury of
     - Transient confusion, disorientation, or impaired consciousness.
     - Dysfunction of memory around the time of injury.
     - Loss or altered state of consciousness lasting less than 30 minutes.
     - Neurological signs (e.g., seizure, dizziness).
   - Mild–complicated TBI includes any of the above *plus* positive neuropathological imaging findings.

2. **What does the cluster symptoms associated with post-concussive syndrome (PCS) look like? These clusters impact each other.**

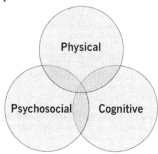

   - Physical symptoms
     - Fatigue, including sleep disturbances.
     - Visual disturbances (eye movement, double vision, blurred vision, light sensitivity).
     - Headaches (slow or sudden).
     - Balance.
     - Nausea.
     - Tinnitus (ringing in ears).
     - Feeling "foggy."
   - Cognitive symptoms
     - Attention—distractibility.
     - Word finding.
     - Slow processing, including listening, reading, writing, and thinking.
     - Memory—new learning, access to information when needed.
     - Executive functions—planning, adjusting, inhibiting, and follow-through.

- Psychosocial symptoms
  - Adjustment to changes in lifestyle; cognitive issues.
  - Injury and symptom validation.
  - Irritability, short fuse.
  - Depression, anxiety.
  - Frustration.

3. **Is there a point where the symptoms from the injury stabilize?** The injury itself evolves over several hours, and changes in the brain may or may not be substantiated immediately after being injured.

   - The majority recover fully within 3–6 weeks of injury.
   - Others take longer (e.g., months to a year) and have permanent symptoms. For these individuals, the *focus is on symptom management* (environmental, schedule changes, or compensatory or new strategies).
   - *Students should be under the care of a medical team* who understand mTBI/concussion and can help them learn to manage their symptoms.

4. **How often should a neuropsychological evaluation be completed? What is the best practice for this?**

   - Many neuropsychological evaluations do not reveal problems students with mTBI have because their problems exist in complex, complicated environments, not in quiet and structured neuropsychological testing situations.
   - Rely also on symptom checklists and compare preinjury to postinjury performance.
   - Best practice is to (a) listen to self-reported symptoms; (b) verify injury with ER report; and (c) believe the students with PCS: most likely they are not making these symptoms and problems up.

5. **What are some of the common impacts you have seen when working with students with PCS?**

   - Students become symptomatic when they have worked (physical and/or mental) too much or too hard.
   - They need regular, frequent intervals of rest (quiet, distraction-free naps).
   - They need to learn to manage their work/effort while managing their symptoms.
   - They get *little to no support* from peers and maybe even family who do not understand their problems when they look "so good." Many show up frustrated, depressed, and doing poorly academically.
   - *They've not done this before,* so (a) they do not know what accommodations they need; (b) they don't know how to advocate for themselves.
   - *They may not even think* that their symptoms are here to stay—there is an evolution of grief that may be delayed.
   - *Trouble keeping up* with class assignments—at first they tend to rely on old habits, then later seek help when they are failing.
   - *Visual problems* result in reading problems that lead to fatigue and/or headaches.
   - *Need new study strategies* based on their unique learning and attention problems.

- *Procrastinating does not work anymore*; they cannot pull it off without having symptoms.
- *Their slow processing* means they need extra time with assignments, exams, and repeating and writing instructions down.
- *They can be easily distracted* in and out of class (e.g., other students tapping pencils during exams becomes unbearable to students with mTBI).
- *They need to adjust their social schedule* in order to prevent fatigue and study more and study differently.

6. **Can you share some experiences about what the recovery process looked like for some of the students you have worked with?**

- When symptoms are managed, when study/organizational strategies are used, when accommodations are provided and used, students can be very successful.
- Students do not know what to expect after injury and operate under their old perceptions of how they studied, learned, and managed their social life. This should change over time as they *experience the impact* of their symptoms on academic life.
- When they are fatigued, it's like running out of gas in your car (e.g., they are suddenly unable to function without rest).
- When first returning or going to college, students with mTBI focus on being successful academically (staying organized, using new study strategies, doing well in courses). As they experience success academically, they begin to focus on relationships with peers (e.g., they cannot drink anymore so new friends are needed, they need more sleep so they cannot party anymore, they need friends who understand and are supportive).

7. **When working with students with PCS, what would be some questions to ask during an intake appointment?**

- Find out if they have attended college postinjury. If so, ask them what they noticed that is different, but *be specific*. Students with mTBI are not always able to retrieve or access all of the information they actually have; this has to do with any number of their symptoms.
- Let their symptoms guide you to ask more specific questions about how their symptoms could affect academics. Some examples are:
  - Fatigue—Do you get tired in 50-minute, 90-minute, and 3-hour classes? What do you do when you get tired? Do you have a place to rest if you can't get home during the day?
  - Light sensitivity—How do you handle bright lights in class? Is there somewhere you can sit that makes lighting easier to handle? Do you wear sunglasses in class and do they help?
  - How do you keep yourself organized? Do you use a smartphone, prompts, timers, campus calendar and planner, Google Calendar, apps, and so forth?
  - What strategies do you use when you read? When you review notes? Do you use large print, text to speech, e-books?

- *Hint:* If students say they're not doing anything different from what they did before their injury, then they are headed into trouble. Confronting them does not get their cooperation. Make sure they know you are there to help, regardless of their willingness to try your suggestions.

8. **What are some challenges disability specialists face when working with students with PCS?**

   - About 50% of these students have had experiences in which health professionals and others have not believed that their symptoms exist. So trust and validation are critical in developing working relationships with them.
   - If physical symptoms become worse, accommodations should change. This is especially important when students first return to college.
   - They are not good advocates, so they need disability services to reach out and provide them with ideas for accommodations.
   - Some do not recognize their challenges and need for accommodation until they have failed.
   - Convincing them to take a reduced load that will allow them to manage symptoms until they see what strategy is going to work or not work.

9. **What are some strategies that you have found to be effective when working with this population?**

   - A college program for students with brain injury, *www.neurocognitivelab.com*: self-learning, self-management, and self-advocacy uses a coaching model. An individualized approach is tailored to each student since each student's injury and symptoms are unique.
     - Supporting them and providing them with advocacy tools since they have not had to be advocates before.
     - Establishing a trusting relationship that validates their symptoms and challenges in college.
     - Learning/study skills and strategies—new learning techniques, rely on outlines or slides ahead of the lecture so they can prepare.
     - Need to record lectures (e.g., with Livescribe [Smartpen]) while they attempt to take notes. Note takers can supplement, but not replace, their own notes.
     - Individualized structure and routine meetings help students develop an inner sense of organization.

10. **What are some assistive technologies that you have found to be useful for accessing print, for staying organized, and for managing time, etc?**

    - Text-to-speech application of a book alongside the paper text.
    - Blinking computer screens or attention-getting visual cues actually compound the visual processing problems many students have. The additional stimulation is stressful and may increase the likelihood of fatigue, especially for students with eye movement disorders. Kurzweil software may not be appropriate.
    - Apps on smartphones, iPhones, iPads, and so forth.

CHAPTER 3

Military Service Members and Veterans in College

Donald L. MacLennan and Leslie Nitta

It is estimated that 2 million veterans may enter U.S. colleges and universities through the use of the post-9/11 GI Bill (Madaus, Miller, & Vance, 2009). The purpose of this chapter, therefore, is to discuss the factors associated with military service that may influence academic performance, with the hope that this information will result in improved methods of coaching military service members and veterans as they enroll in college. The specific objectives of this chapter include:

- Describe the complex pattern of injuries and symptoms associated with military service and combat deployment that may influence a service member's/veteran's return to school.

- Facilitate an appreciation of military culture that may enhance communication with service members and veterans and support development of a strong therapeutic alliance.

BLASTS, TBI, AND THE WOUNDS OF WAR

The wars in Afghanistan (Operation Enduring Freedom [OEF]) and Iraq (Operation Iraqi Freedom [OIF]) and the withdrawal phase of Operation New Dawn

Leslie Nitta, MA, CCC-SLP, Department of Speech Pathology, Greater Los Angeles Veterans Administration Healthcare System, Los Angeles, California

Donald L. MacLennan, MS, CCC-SLP, Speech Pathology Section, Minneapolis Veterans Administration Medical Center, Minneapolis, Minnesota

(OND) represent the longest military engagements in U.S. history. Since 2001, an estimated 2.7 million service members have been deployed to Iraq and Afghanistan (Watson Institute for International and Public Affairs, 2015), with more than 1.6 million service members transitioning to veteran status (Adams, 2013). These wars have been characterized by enemy use of explosive devices, resulting in a high incidence of blast exposure among service members and veterans. Over half of all injuries sustained in combat are associated with explosive devices (Hoge et al., 2008; Terrio et al., 2009). Blasts may result in primary injuries related to pressurization waves. Other injuries may be associated with flying debris, falls, and fumes or toxins associated with the blast wave (Warden, 2006). Improvements in protective military gear and battlefield medicine have effectively increased the probability of surviving these injuries, which may include TBI. As in the civilian population, 75–90% of the TBIs sustained in Iraq and Afghanistan are of mild severity (Hoge et al., 2008; Schell & Marshall, 2008; Terrio et al., 2009). The Defense and Veterans Brain Injury Center (DVBIC, 2015) reports that there were 320,344 TBIs sustained in the military worldwide between 2000 and 2014 by both deployed and nondeployed service members. Of these TBIs, 82.5% were classified as mild, 8.3% as moderate, 1% as severe, 1.4% as penetrating brain injuries, and 6.8% as not classifiable. Iverson, Langlois, McCrea, and Kelly (2009) note that the total number of reported TBIs may include both false-positive and false-negative reports due to a screening method that was designed to capture as many TBIs as possible. These totals reflect the number of individuals *who reported TBI(s)*, not the number of individuals who continue to be symptomatic. Other challenges in identifying mild TBI in military personnel include screenings that occur long after an event and the inclusion of individuals who reported being "dazed and confused" as a natural reaction to the stress of combat (Iverson, 2010; MacGregor, Dougherty, Tang, & Galarneau, 2012).

While moderate to severe TBI is commonly associated with significant cognitive challenges in attention, memory, and executive functions, mild TBI (also known as *concussion*) is typically associated with an excellent prognosis. Evidence from the civilian population and athletes (Iverson, 2005; McCrea et al., 2003; McCrory et al., 2013) suggest that the vast majority of these individuals experience resolution of neuropsychological symptoms within 3 months postinjury. Some individuals do, however, report persistent post-concussion symptoms, the prevalence of which is reported to range from 2 to more than 20% in the civilian population (e.g., Alves, Macciocchi, & Barth, 1993; Gunstad & Suhr, 2004; Wood, 2007). Numerous studies have indicated that chronic post-concussion symptoms in service members and veterans are more likely to be associated with comorbid conditions such as PTSD than with mild TBI (e.g., Hoge et al., 2008; Polusny et al., 2011). Regardless of etiology, persistent cognitive difficulties in this population can undermine college performance.

Some service members and veterans with a history of mild TBI report persistent cognitive impairments in areas of concentration and memory years after injury. Professionals should be aware that mild TBI is not synonymous with post-concussion syndrome. Combat experiences may contribute to physical or psychological difficulties that may persist well beyond the period of deployment (Belanger, Donnell, & Vanderploeg, 2014). It should also be noted that deployment to a war zone can contribute to neuropsychological compromise even in the absence of a brain injury. Vasterling and colleagues (2006) found that deployed individuals demonstrated reduced performance on measures of sustained attention and memory, suggesting that combat deployment *itself* is associated with subtle alterations of neural functioning.

Posttraumatic Stress Disorder

Since the beginning of the war in Afghanistan in 2001, combat-deployed service members and veterans have been diagnosed with PTSD, chronic pain, and TBI, a group of conditions that have been referred to as the "polytrauma clinical triad" (Lew et al., 2009). Brain trauma and combat stress were observed as early as World War I because of German use of explosives on artillery shells; the condition was labeled "shell shock" or "neuroasthenia" (Shively & Perl, 2012). During World War II and the Korean War, service members exhibiting anxiety, depression, mood swings, sleep disturbance, substance abuse, and suicidality were diagnosed with "combat fatigue" or "battle fatigue."

The American Psychiatric Association established this cluster of symptoms as PTSD in 1980, 5 years after the end of the Vietnam conflict. PTSD is tied to exposure to an etiological event (or events) that involve the threat of death or serious injury and results in significant distress or impairment of an individual's social interactions, capacity to work, or ability to function in other important areas (American Psychiatric Association, 2013). Hoge and colleagues (2004) found that 12.2–12.9% soldiers and Marines deployed to Iraq and 6.2% of those deployed to Afghanistan met diagnostic criteria for PTSD 3–4 months postdeployment. PTSD is an *anxiety disorder* characterized by reexperiencing of a feeling, thought, or event; avoidance behaviors; changes in arousal and reactivity; and persistent negative changes in cognitions and mood (American Psychiatric Association, 2013). Diagnostic criteria for PTSD include, but are not limited to, sleep disturbance, irritability, aggressive behavior, hypervigilance, concentration problems, and an exaggerated startle response (American Psychiatric Association, 2013).

In a study that compared Operation Desert Storm veterans with and without PTSD, Vasterling, Brailey, Constans, and Sutker (1998) found that neurocognitive findings in the PTSD group included, but were not limited to, mild deficits in the areas of sustained attention possibly associated with disordered arousal, but no deficits in selective or shifting attention. Regarding memory, deficiencies were noted in working memory and/or mental manipulation of information and in initial acquisition of information but there was no deficit for retention of learned information. The PTSD group also experienced more interference from previously presented information during learning tasks, as indicated by higher error rates, and greater difficulty in separating relevant and irrelevant information than the non-PTSD group.

Vasterling and Brailey's (2005) literature review found that individuals with initiation problems possibly associated with prefrontal lobe dysfunction engage in less spontaneous strategy generation, although they may successfully use strategies after some instruction. This finding suggests that these individuals may not require extensive services to support strategy use after initial instruction. Vasterling and Brailey also discuss cognitive dysfunction as a by-product of not being fully engaged, that is, disconnected from activities that require their full potential. While it is beyond the scope of this chapter to summarize the PTSD literature, it is important for any professional who works with combat-deployed individuals to appreciate that PTSD can result in symptoms that are similar to those of post-concussion syndrome.

Chronic Pain

Pain is a complicated phenomenon. Acute pain alerts one to possible injury. Chronic pain, however, may persist beyond an acute injury and *in the absence* of a past injury or evidence of physical damage (American Academy of Pain Medicine, n.d., *www.painmed.org/patientcenter/facts-on-pain/#chronic*). In a retrospective study of 340 OEF/OIF veterans from Department of Veterans Affairs (VA) medical centers, 81.5% reported chronic pain, with back pain (58%) and headache pain (55%) being the most common (Lew et al., 2009). Because headache pain is frequently reported by veterans with concomitant PTSD and a history of mild TBI or more severe TBI, professionals may be tempted to attribute headache to brain injury. However, there is a possibility that headaches may not be associated with a *single* etiology; headaches "are unique among pain conditions in their degree of responsiveness to combined medical and psychological intervention" (Borkum, 2007, p. 3). Regardless of etiology, headaches and pain in general are cause for concern. Von Korff, Dworkin, Le Resche, and Kruger (1988) found that individuals with headache and back pain reported higher activity limitations than those with other pain conditions, and that pain was associated with psychological distress.

Sleep Disorders

A secondary factor influencing the cognitive and daily functioning of OEF/OIF/OND veterans is sleep dysfunction. Sleep problems are included among the diagnostic criteria of multiple mental health disorders that include, but are not limited to, PTSD, major depressive disorder, and generalized anxiety disorder (American

Psychiatric Association, 2013). Sleep problems can be classified as total sleep deprivation and partial sleep deprivation. Partial sleep deprivation is categorized as sleep fragmentation, selective sleep stage deprivation, and reduced sleep duration (Banks & Dinges, 2007). In a prospective study in which sleep was restricted to 4–6 hours per night for 14 days, performance on cognitive tasks that assess working memory and sustained attention were comparable to that of individuals who were completely deprived of sleep for 1–2 days (Van Dongen, Maislin, Mullington, & Dinges, 2003). Mysliwiec and colleagues (2013) found that 41.8% of service members with combat experience reported 5 hours or less of sleep per night. Luxton and colleagues (2011) found that short sleep duration is common and persists in redeployed soldiers in the postdeployment period. Reasons for reduced sleep include disturbing dreams (Troxel et al., 2015), pain, and inability to slow thoughts (Polley, Frank, & Smith, 2012). Poor sleep is a concern because individuals with insomnia symptoms prior to deployment have been found to be at higher risk for new onset of PTSD, depression, and anxiety following deployment (Gehrman et al., 2013) and future suicidal ideation (Ribeiro et al., 2012).

Depression and Moral Injury

Hoge and colleagues (2004) found that 14–15% of Army soldiers reported symptoms associated with depression after deployment in Afghanistan and Iraq when questioned 3–4 months postdeployment. The literature generally reveals that both PTSD and depression are experienced by a large number of those who served in combat in Iraq and Afghanistan, and that the prevalence of both conditions increase as the time since returning from deployment increases (Tanelian & Jaycox, 2008).

Katon, Kleinman, and Rosen (1982) describe depression as a "biopsychosocial illness with characteristic biologic or vegetative symptoms, psychological changes in affect and cognition and often antecedent social stressors as well as consequences for the social support system as a result of the illness" (pp. 245–246). Symptoms of major depressive disorder and major depressive episodes (MDD/MDE) include, but are not limited to, insomnia or hypersomnia, fatigue, observable psychomotor agitation or retardation, feelings of worthlessness or inappropriate guilt, diminished ability to think or concentrate, more indecisiveness, and recurrent thoughts of death or suicide (American Psychiatric Association, 2013). Furthermore, it is important to note that MDD/MDE symptoms overlap with those of post-concussion syndrome as well as those for generalized anxiety disorder, for which DSM-5 (American Psychiatric Association, 2013) criteria include, but are not limited to, restlessness, being easily fatigued, difficulty concentrating, irritability, and sleep disturbance. It is also worth noting that depression is one of the most common causes of somatization (Katon et al., 1982), which is associated with increased utilization of medical care (Katon, Berg, Robins, & Risse, 1986).

Taken at face value, it is not surprising that some individuals who participate in combat may experience depression and anxiety; war is characterized by death and destruction. Beyond physical and psychological injuries, increasing attention is being paid to moral injury, a condition that results in ethical and moral distress (Litz et al., 2009). In his book *War and the Soul,* Edward Tick (2005) cites Erik Erikson's comments about a "central disturbance . . . of ego identity" in his veteran patients that resulted in disrupted cohesion; their lives appeared to no longer hang together (p. 105). As professionals, we have often heard veterans describe this loss of cognitive continuity through comments expressing their perceptions of current functioning (e.g., "I can't remember anything anymore"). The comment "I used to remember *everything*" is also occasionally heard from individuals with a history of concussion/mild TBI. This comment may reflect a tendency to overestimate past performance and attribute all symptoms to a negative event, a phenomenon referred to as the "good-old-days bias" (Gundstad & Suhr, 2001; Lange, Iverson, & Rose, 2010). Of interest, these individuals often report excellent cognitive performance throughout deployment with cognitive deterioration occurring only after returning home. Although coaches cannot directly address moral and ethical distress, they can refer individuals to a mental health provider and can help an individual develop a "student" identity through coaching that supports increasing self-efficacy for academic activities.

Substance Use

Given the previous description of conditions that may be experienced by service members and veterans, their high rate of substance use may not be surprising. Graham and Cardon (2008) surveyed OEF/OIF veterans and found that of those who screened positive for both PTSD and a prior TBI, 65.9% reported past alcohol use and 53% reported current alcohol use. Because of the relatively common co-occurrence of TBI, substance use disorder, and PTSD, Najavits, Highley, Dolan, and Fee (2012) refer to the triad as a "trimorbid disorder" with symptoms that include, but are not limited to, deficits in attention, concentration, and delayed memory; disinhibition; and lack of insight.

Misattribution of Symptoms and Iatrogenesis

It is important to note that physicians and other medical providers (e.g., a physiatrist, neurologist, neuropsychologist, and neurobehaviorist) diagnose and attribute symptoms of concussion; these professionals are trained to interpret a broad range of evaluation findings that include effort testing and neuroimaging. Misdiagnosis can occur because of the overlap of post-concussion symptoms with other conditions such as depression. For example, Iverson (2006) found that 9 out of 10 depressed individuals met liberal criteria and 5 out of 10 met conservative criteria for PCS likely because "perceived cognitive impairment is a cardinal feature of depression" (p. 304).

When providing psychoeducation addressing cognitive symptoms after mild TBI, professionals need to be mindful of the potential to cause long-lasting harm due to misattribution of symptoms (e.g., Hoge, Goldberb, & Castro, 2009). Mittenberg, DiGulio, Perrin, and Bass (1992) theorized that a cycle of symptom reinforcement may contribute to an expectation of persistence of symptoms. Interested readers are referred to Roth and Spencer (2013), who describe an example of iatrogenesis in an Iraq war veteran with a history of mild TBI who reported "severe" or "very severe" cognitive problems.

CONSIDERING THE MILITARY CULTURE IN AN EDUCATIONAL CONTEXT

Military Culture and Battlemind

Military culture is defined by Exum, Coll, and Weiss (2011) as the "values, beliefs, traditions, norms, perceptions and behaviors that govern how members of the armed forces think, communicate and interact with one another as well as with civilians" (p. 17). The principles instilled in military culture are intended to guide the behavior of service members throughout their lives both on and off duty (Coll, Weiss, & Yarvis, 2010).

The primary function of the military is combat (Dunivin, 1994). Each branch of military service has a unique but overlapping set of values intended to foster cohesive, highly disciplined units that can reliably carry out combat missions. Values related to honor, integrity, and loyalty are found in all branches of military service and ensure that service members are truthful and adhere to strict principles of moral conduct. Courage, commitment, and devotion to duty are values that enable service members to find the strength to complete their missions in the face of hardship, adversity, and mortal danger. These values help foster group cohesion and trust in which there is the expectation that service members will make sacrifices for the greater good (Hooker, 2003). They also foster much-needed group interdependence needed to complete complex missions. Military values emphasize discipline and motivation to succeed. One student attributed his academic success to his military experience by stating that "the first [time] I ever met my drill sergeant in training, he told my platoon that the only things we would need to succeed are discipline and motivation" (Ness, Rocke, Harrist, & Vroman, 2014, p. 154). Other student veterans reported that their military experience and values had a positive impact on their academic careers in areas such as self-motivation, ability to prioritize tasks, and effectively manage their time (Ness et al., 2014; Rumann & Hamrick,

2010). Thus, some military traits and values related to discipline and commitment may have a positive impact on self-regulatory skills critical to academic success.

Battlemind training refers to skills and behaviors that are taught to service members to support their combat experience and ensure their survival (Castro, 2006). These skills are adaptive in a theater of combat in that they serve to enhance the safety of service members as well as the success of combat missions. Potential problems arise when these combat skill sets become "hardwired" and remain active after deployment. Table 3.1 includes aspects of battlemind and describes

TABLE 3.1. Aspects of Battlemind and How These Relate to the College Experiences of Service Member and Veteran Students

Combat	Civilian context
Tactical awareness versus hypervigilance	
Survival is contingent on acute awareness of the combat environment. Service members are taught to develop a 360-degree sphere of vigilance to ensure their safety.	Service members and veterans may feel anxious, particularly in large groups or confined spaces where there is a poor "line of sight" to detect a threat and few avenues of escape. This anxiety may contribute to distractibility. Service members and veterans have learned to divide attention across many aspects of their environment, whereas a civilian context may require selective attention with a specific focus. Individuals with recent combat experience may be smiling and attentive during an interview, but when questioned, their thoughts may have been somewhere else, related to a noise they heard or a movement they saw out the window. Such inattention may affect concentration for lectures and homework assignments.
Targeted versus inappropriate aggression	
Combat is a stressful environment where split-second decisions impact whether one will "kill or be killed." Anger is a weapon that keeps the service member alert, awake, and focused.	Heightened irritability and anger may be a barrier against social relationships. Service members and veterans may misinterpret what others say and overreact to intended humor or minor insults.
Mission OPSEC (Operation Security) versus secretiveness	
Discussion of missions in a combat theater is on a need-to-know basis so as not to jeopardize the security of the mission. Implicit in this is that, in theater, you confide in only the people whom you trust.	Service members and veterans may be reluctant to share combat experiences with others, even as they pertain to conditions that serve as barriers to college performance.
Buddies (cohesion) versus withdrawal	
Service members and veterans may be slow to trust professionals in rehabilitation or college settings without combat experience who haven't "been there, done that." Service members/veterans' battle buddies are like family whom they could trust with their lives.	Service members and veterans may prefer to be with other combat veterans who, consequently, limit the range of social experiences available to them on campus.

how they may relate to the college experiences of the service member/veteran student.

The goal of the professional providing support services to service members and veterans is to develop military cultural competence, or the ability to understand and appreciate military culture so as to better engage and provide rehabilitation and academic support to individuals with a military background. Some examples of how an appreciation of military culture can enhance services for this group include the following.

Incorporating Military Service and Values in an Interview by Being Prepared and Knowledgeable and by Understanding Rank and Occupation

- *Be prepared.* Some service members and veterans have difficulty establishing trust with civilians; one way to convey a sincere desire to help is to have the fullest possible knowledge of their military experience. In our practice, we perform a thorough chart review prior to the initial interview, present our understanding of the service member's/veteran's history, and invite confirmation or correction of the information. We ask if there is anything else that would be helpful for us to know. If a military history is unavailable, it may be helpful to acquire information during the initial conversation. Coll, Weiss, and Yarvis (2010) provide a list of suggested questions to begin the interview, including:

>"In which branch of the armed forces did you serve?"
>
>"Where were you stationed?"
>
>"What was your military occupational specialty [MOS]?"
>
>"Do you have any family or friends who are still deployed?"
>
>"Were you engaged in combat?"

- *Be knowledgeable.* Use correct terminology when addressing a service member. The term "soldier" applies only to military personnel serving in the army. Calling a member of the Marines a soldier may inadvertently offend some individuals. Marines prefer to call themselves "marines." Members of the navy may prefer the term "sailor," and members of the Air Force may prefer the term "airman." The term "service member" is a generic term that can apply to people serving in all branches of military service.

- *Understand military rank structure and occupational performance.* Estimates of preinjury cognitive skills may be inferred from information related to achievement of developmental milestones, academic history, and vocational history as well as best performance on evaluation test measures (Lezak, Howieson, Bigler, & Tranel, 2012). Knowledge of military rank and responsibilities associated with that rank are essential to reliably evaluate vocational history. Individuals deployed in military service may have helped in the governance of villages and cities by setting up hospitals, building roads, and opening schools. They may have coordinated operations involving air and ground units with little margin for error. They may have been asked to solve complex problems under highly challenging conditions (Shinseki, 2013). It is wise to consider that service members and veterans bring a depth of life experience to college endeavors that may compensate for the learning difficulties that they may report and/or demonstrate.

Being Aware of Factors That May Cause Stress for a Service Member

The military places high value on punctuality. In combat, lives may be lost if troops or materials arrive late. Service members and veterans often use the phrase "If you're not early, you're late." It is not uncommon in the context of rehabilitation for providers to start a session late or to hold a patient past his or her scheduled time. Providers without appreciation of military culture may have no idea of the stress this imposes on some service members and veterans who have either been waiting for the provider to show up or are now late for the next appointment. The provider who understands the importance of punctuality in military culture is more likely to start and complete sessions on time, or at least ask permission to extend the session when necessary.

Adjusting Services in Subtle Ways to Allow Service Members to Reach Goals

Service members who have sustained an injury such as a TBI will, at some point, receive a medical evaluation, or "Med Board," to determine fitness for return to duty. When beginning services with active duty service members, we ask how they would like to be addressed. Most often, they choose to be addressed informally on a first-name basis. We then ask how they would like to be addressed in the medical record; addressing them by rank in the medical record (e.g., "SSG" or "Staff Sergeant Smith" instead of "John" or "Mr. Smith") might reinforce their intention to return to duty and may subtly influence healthcare providers who review their files. In our experience, many service members with strong aspirations to return to duty choose to be addressed by rank in the medical record.

The Need for Supports for Veterans and Service Members in College

As of 2012 over 945,000 college students in the United States had a military affiliation that provided eligibility to receive benefits under the Post-9/11 GI Bill (Kirkwood,

2014). While some research raises concerns regarding the attrition rate of veterans in college (Ness & Vroman, 2014), a recent study by the Student Veterans of America (SVA) indicated that over half the veterans receiving benefits from the GI Bill are attaining degrees (Jelinek, 2014). However, there are indications that veterans, especially those who have experienced combat, have challenges that make it more difficult for them to meet the expectations of college than their nonmilitary, nondeployed counterparts. The SVA study reported that, while the graduation rate for veterans (51.7%) was slightly less than that for nonveteran traditional students (56%), it took them longer to achieve this milestone; the majority of veteran students in this study completed an associate's degree within 4 years and an undergraduate degree within 6 years. Barriers to completing college may include interruptions related to deployments for students serving in the National Guard and Army Reserve, as well as the possible impact of a history of mild TBI and multiple comorbidities on the ability to navigate the college experience, integrate into campus life, and successfully meet the academic demands. There is also evidence, however, that there are strengths developed through their military training that help them to meet those challenges.

The motivation to apply to college is often based on both intrinsic and extrinsic factors (Ness et al., 2014). The lure of financial aid for school can be a powerful incentive for veterans who have recently demobilized or separated from the military and have no income. However, this incentive to enroll can backfire if deployment-related factors result in poor school performance because the funds associated with the Post-9/11 GI Bill are contingent on acceptable academic achievement. Veterans may be required to pay back education benefits if they fail in school. This underscores the importance of developing support services for veterans that maximize their chances for success.

Grossman (2009) outlined the difficulties and needs of service members and veterans seeking to enter college and extended a challenge to U.S. colleges and universities to prepare for what he described as a "perfect storm." First, the Americans with Disabilities Act Amendment Act of 2008 (ADAAA) makes it easier to qualify for cognitive disability. In addition, the ADAAA removes exclusionary criteria for cognitive disability, which allows people with disabilities to maintain services under the law even if they are receiving treatment for their disability (e.g., previously a person with concentration difficulty who was taking Ritalin may have been denied disability services in the belief that the pharmacological treatment would have effectively mitigated the impact of the cognitive impairment). Second, the passage in July 2008 of the Post-9/11 GI Bill expanded the range of educational assistance services. For those who qualify, the Post-9/11 GI Bill can provide full tuition and fees, a monthly housing allowance, and up to $1,000 a year for books and supplies while attending school. Third, these education bills are having a significant impact on enrollment of veterans in colleges and universities, including those with medical, mental health, and cognitive challenges stemming from their histories of TBI and comorbid conditions associated with military service. Grossman proposed that colleges provide service members and veterans with campus champions, who understand the complex nature of their injuries and can help them access the services they require to successfully perform at the college level and graduate with a degree that will translate into a meaningful career.

College campuses are faced with a number of challenges that may complicate how disability services are provided to meet the academic and counseling needs of the combat service member and veteran. Simply identifying candidates for disability services may be problematic. Service members and veterans may be less likely to self-identify for disability services because they may be unaware of the "rights and responsibilities" of students who meet the criteria for disability services (Madaus et al., 2009) and/or they may be reluctant to acknowledge difficulties (Shackelford, 2009) due to a "warrior strength" cultural value (Dunivin, 1994). Moreover, college personnel may have difficulty identifying disabilities in service member/veteran students because the psychological, emotional, and cognitive difficulties associated with deployment-related conditions are often "hidden" (Madaus et al., 2009).

Vance and Miller (2009) surveyed members of the Association on Higher Education and Disabilities regarding the needs of combat service members and veterans and found that respondents identified multiple sources of disability. Services provided to these students focused most frequently on psychological and emotional issues related to conditions like PTSD, followed by health and medical issues such as pain or impairments in vision and/or hearing, then learning disability related to cognitive impairments. Respondents to the Vance and Miller survey indicated that the highest demand for services was in the area of academic services (e.g., tutoring and writing labs), followed by curricular adjustments (e.g., life credits, veterans-only classes), career counseling (e.g., transferring military experience to civilian vocations), and academic adjustments (e.g., priority registration, academic accommodations). Like Grossman (2009), Madaus and colleagues (2009) strongly recommend that college campus programs provide veterans with services staff familiar with the unique needs of veterans. They also recommend that campus programs collaborate with VA programs.

A number of studies have investigated the influence of deployment, TBI, and/ or PTSD on the college performance of veterans (Ellison et al., 2012; Ness et al., 2014; Rumann & Hamrick, 2010; Smee, Buenrostro, Garrick, Sreenivasan, & Weinberger, 2013). These studies revealed common themes across areas related to educational planning, military culture and social relationships, effects of hyperarousal and anxiety, and cognitive challenges, all of which are summarized in the following sections.

Educational Planning and Navigating College Life

Service member and veteran students reported a need for easy access to comprehensive academic counseling due to their lack of familiarity with admission procedures, financial aid options, campus services, enrollment procedures, and degree planning. One student indicated he had moved across the country to enroll in a college that offered enhanced veteran services that he had discovered, by chance, while conducting an Internet search (Ellison et al., 2012). Other study participants reported difficulties in completing tasks and often identified a strong reluctance to disclose their disability and seek help, factors that may undermine the complex process of applying for school, obtaining financial aid, developing an academic plan, and fulfilling class requirements (Smee et al., 2013). Some student veterans reported a history of academic difficulties and a greater need for supportive services. As one of them said, "Let's face it, many of these guys went into the service because they were no good at school" (Ellison et al., p. 212). Younger veterans may desire more support and guidance, while older veterans often had clear occupational and academic goals in mind and required less assistance in educational planning.

Some difficulties navigating college life may stem from drastic changes inherent in transitioning from a military to civilian setting. Military life is highly structured; there are few choices regarding what to wear, when to eat, and when and where to work. Decision making in the military is based on a clear chain of command, and student veterans indicated that they had become accustomed to being told what to do. During deployments, tasks are set up and are repeatedly practiced until they become routine (Rumann & Hamrick, 2010). Some student veterans acknowledged challenges in adapting to an educational environment that provides little in the way of structure and routine and the requirement to make many more decisions (Ness et al., 2014). In addition, the demands of school are often more time-intensive than a military workload as the GI Bill requires students to take a nearly full-time courseload, and classes require many hours of work outside of class time.

Ellison and colleagues (2012) point out that some younger veterans who have gone directly from high school into military service may never have developed the basic life skills that support the ability to live independently. Postdeployment problems related to medical and psychosocial stressors amplify the difficulties associated with the military-to-school transition and can result in a downward life trajectory that includes "homelessness, disintegrating family support, urgent clinical needs such as addiction relapses, physical injury and disability" (p. 212). Many veterans choose not to live with their family and endure financial hardships associated with paying for suitable housing, transportation needs, and bills, while trying to find the time and resources to commit to a demanding school schedule. One survey respondent reported knowing several veterans who became overwhelmed by the combined stressors of financial obligations and demands of school, resulting in depression and substance use and, ultimately, dropped out of college.

Military Culture and Social Relationships

Military culture fosters the camaraderie of service members as successful combat missions require a high degree of interdependence and trust. Accustomed to tight social bonds during military service, many veterans report feeling lonely and isolated in the comparatively less organized social structure on campus (Ness et al., 2014). Veteran students report "feeling invisible" and may have a difficult time developing relationships with other students and faculty. Rumann and Hamrick (2010) comment that veterans returning from combat perceive themselves as having matured in ways that student peers have not. Student veterans also report feelings of annoyance with peers who become upset by minor everyday events that seem trivial in comparison to the life-threatening experiences of combat. Some veterans expressed frustration due to the perceived substandard work ethic demonstrated by their nonveteran student peers. Civilian students sometimes ask such insensitive questions as "Did you kill anyone?" or "Did you see anyone get blown up?" These types of questions typically provoke annoyance, which may be compounded by issues with irritability and anger that many report experiencing in the first year back from combat (Ness et al., 2014; Rumann & Hamrick, 2010; Smee et al., 2013).

Respondents in most surveys indicated it was easier to socialize with other veterans, often reporting an inherent trust in other veterans who have experienced combat (Ellison et al., 2012). Shared experiences, the ability to communicate using the unique language and humor of their military culture, and an appreciation of the challenges involved in transitioning to civilian life were also cited as factors that contributed to socializing among veterans (Rumann & Hamrick, 2010). Ellison and colleagues (2012) observe that both young and older veterans expressed a need for peer support from veterans who have "been there" to overcome problems related to postdeployment adjustment and transition to school.

Hyperarousal and Anxiety

Hyperarousal and concerns for safety occur for a variety of reasons in many service members and veterans after deployment, and they are especially prominent in those with PTSD. These stress responses are normal and functional behaviors for a warrior in a combat setting; however, they can become accidentally triggered in a civilian context (Hoge, 2010). Veteran students in the surveys under discussion frequently identified the presence of hypervigilance, particularly in areas of the campus with high levels of noise and activity (Ness et al., 2014), in the event of a sudden loud noise, or in the presence of road construction, which was often the location of roadside bombs in theater of combat (Ellison et al., 2012). One student described "people rushing by you" as a trigger for a safety reaction; he reported that part of his brain was always performing a threat analysis. Many respondents shared a similar discomfort when people walked behind them (Rumann & Hamrick, 2010).

Students cope with hyperarousal and safety concerns in a variety of ways, some positive and others negative. Some students sit in the back of the class from where they have a "line of sight" to monitor the entire classroom. This may conflict with recommended compensatory cognitive strategies, such as the frequent recommendation to sit in front of the class to decrease distraction. Other standard strategies used as cognitive supports also may be used as compensation for anxiety as well. For example, proctored exams may be given in a distraction-free environment with additional time allowance (Ellison et al., 2012), an accommodation that is also appropriate for slowed cognitive processing. Students also reported withdrawing to a quiet place on campus (Ness et al., 2014) or using substances to help alleviate their stress and anxiety.

Cognitive Challenges

Given the difficulties reported by student veterans who have served in combat, it is interesting that they did not identify cognitive symptoms as a significant barrier to academic activities in a study by Ness and colleagues (2012). In a larger sample of veteran students, some with a history of TBI or current symptoms of PTSD, study subjects described "robust academic achievement" (Ness & Vroman, 2014).

The most interesting finding was that while students with a history of TBI and/or a current diagnosis of PTSD showed lower scores of self-efficacy for learning than students without a history of TBI and/or current PTSD symptomatology, their GPAs did not differ. This is surprising, as academic self-efficacy is typically a strong predictor of GPA (Zajacova, Lynch, & Espenshade, 2005). While the authors indicate this result might be partially accounted for by sampling bias, there may be another explanation. Military culture promotes a strong work ethic, characterized by self-discipline, punctuality, and self-sufficiency. There is evidence that these qualities may provide some measure of resiliency that allows some student veterans to achieve academic success despite a perception of reduced academic self-efficacy. Military service and particularly deployment experience was credited by respondents as providing them with a maturity and clearer perspective on life that motivated them to engage in school and a confidence that they would be able to successfully meet the challenges they faced (Rumann & Hamrick, 2010). One respondent stated, "Don't worry, you know, you can't do anything in college that's as challenging as your first week at basic training as a 17-year-old, or your first couple of months of deployment, or that first 25-mile road march you gotta go on" (Ness et al., 2014, p. 154). The process of internalizing motivation and discipline begins during basic training and is reinforced throughout the military experience (Rumann & Hamrick, 2010). When applied to an academic setting, student veterans indicated that motivation and discipline helped them get to class, study, and complete term papers. As one veteran described it, "In the combat zone, it's life threatening not to do your job" (Ness et al., 2014, p. 154). Students in both studies credited their military experience with making them better students than they were prior to enlistment. These studies indicate that overall self-efficacy may be heightened by military experience to a degree that may allow service member/ veteran students to succeed in school despite reduced academic self-efficacy.

Smee and colleagues (2013) encourage college coaches who work with service members and veterans to present accommodations as "resilience builders" that enhance cognitive strengths rather than "compensate" for weaknesses. This approach aligns with the military "warrior strength" model and promotes positive expectations for success. They recommend appealing to military values by challenging students to be active learners and to take leadership roles in the classroom and adapting military procedures to the academic arena. For example, successful mission planning and execution rely on the same steps and skills as college participation: organization of schedules and materials; development of and adherence to timelines; development of skills through repetition, effort, and diligence; and knowledge that one's strengths and use of accommodations to compensate for one's weaknesses will result in successful completion of a college program. Most important, service members and veterans are accustomed to an "after-action review" following a mission during which they determine what went right, what went wrong, and what would be done differently during the next mission. Students may be encouraged to use after-action reviews to self-evaluate current study practices and the effectiveness of accommodations. These skills are highly consistent with the self-regulatory practices inherent in dynamic coaching.

A SUMMARY OF RECOMMENDATIONS FOR POSTSECONDARY SETTINGS

1. *Provide a wide array of available supports.* Service members and veterans will present with varying needs. Many will require no supports at all. Others may require supports extending far beyond academic accommodations to include medical and mental health services, substance abuse counseling, and rehabilitation. Some may require services to help them access appropriate supports and resources to address crises related to financial hardship, homelessness, and family conflict.

Students may require counselor advocates who can work on a 1:1 basis to guide them through basic processes associated with college application and enrollment procedures and navigating a college system. The fullest range of academic accommodations should be available to meet the needs of these wounded warriors transitioning back into the community.

2. *Provide education to college faculty and college administrative staff.* Education should focus on military culture, the natural history of mild TBI, the consequences of TBI for some students, and how conditions commonly associated with combat may influence academic performance. A full understanding of these issues may help college staff identify students who are in need of support services and provide them with a sensitivity that may decrease the stigmatization that these students may feel. There should be guidance on the inherent dangers of misattributing post-concussion symptoms to mild TBI that may result in the development of persisting cognitive symptoms that would otherwise resolve. Specific instruction on creating positive expectations for recovery and building resilience may be especially helpful in this regard.

3. *Support the development of veterans' organizations and activities on campus.* Veterans' organizations can provide an avenue for socialization, validation of the rewards and challenges associated with military service and deployments, and peer support for the life challenges these students are experiencing.

4. *Partner with the VA to provide the fullest range of expert services.* The VA's polytrauma system of care provides a wide range of medical, mental health, and rehabilitation programs that can help manage the complex needs of combat veterans (U.S. Department of Veterans Affairs, 2015). The VA can be a resource for accommodations that involve a monetary cost. For example, assistive technology for cognition may be provided free to eligible veterans. Mental health and rehabilitation services may be provided across great distances through telehealth connections to community-based outpatient clinics or veterans' homes. Postsecondary staff are encouraged to develop relationships with case managers within mental health and rehabilitation programs for guidance regarding access to services. Recent VA grants have made it possible to increase the VA's presence on campus to provide direct support to veterans through programs such as VITAL (see VA Campus Toolkit under Additional Resources).

ADDITIONAL RESOURCES

- For more information on mild TBI and/or PTSD, readers are referred to Cifu and Blake (2011), Vasterling, Verfaelllie, and Sullivan (2009), and Vasterling, Bryant, and Keane (2012).

- For more information on military culture, readers are referred to *Once a Warrior, Always a Warrior* (Hoge, 2010).

- For practical information on selecting and financing college and helping veterans get back to school, coaches are referred to "Back to School Guide to Academic Success after Traumatic Brain Injury" (*http://dvbic.dcoe.mil/back-school-guide-academic-success-after-traumatic-brain-injury*).

- The VA Campus Toolkit is a community engagement initiative designed to assist student veterans to meet their educational goals through collaborative efforts with higher education institutions, on-campus clinical therapy, and care management services (*www.mentalhealth.va.gov/studentveteran/#sthash.A27Wvw1s.dpbs*).

- The Warrior Scholar Project consists of immersive 1- and 2-week academic workshops or "bootcamps" provided free of charge to enlisted veterans and are held at some of America's top colleges and universities (*http://warrior-scholar.org/about.html*).

- "Understanding the Effects of Concussion, Blast, and Brain Injuries: A Guide for Families, Veterans, and Caregivers" is an online guide to help support families, veterans, caregivers, and therapists with service members who have sustained TBIs (*www.brainlinemilitary.org/content/2008/11/understanding-effects-concussion-blast-and-brain-injuries-guide-families-veterans-and-caregi_pageall.html*).

- For more information on working with service members and veterans in the workplace, home, and college, see a recent publication by the Department of Defense, Department of Veterans Affairs, and experts on TBI, *A Clinician's Guide to Cognitive Rehabilitation in mild TBI: An Application to Military Service Members and Veterans* (Mashima et al., 2017).

- If a veteran is suicidal, professionals should immediately connect him or her with a mental health provider and/or a suicide prevention coordinator. Community providers can defer to the Veterans Crisis Line at 1-800-273-8255 and press 1, or text 838255 to get help immediately.

PART II
DYNAMIC COACHING

CHAPTER 4

A Dynamic Coaching Approach

Nearly everyone, at one time or another, has had experience with coaches. Maybe you've been coached or maybe you've even been an athletic coach. Merriam-Webster's dictionary defines a "coach" as a person who teaches and trains an athlete or performer; teaches and trains the members of a sports team and makes decisions about how the team plays during games; or gives someone lessons in a particular subject. There are many kinds of coaches who instruct and support individuals for a wide range of activities. For example, there are voice coaches for singers and "life" coaches for individuals seeking direction in achieving a personal or career goal. Regardless of the purpose, coaching involves teaching or instructing. What coaches teach, how they teach, when they teach, and where they teach will vary depending on the individual, the context, and the purpose.

In this chapter, I provide an overview of our coaching approach and its critical elements, and start by addressing the question Who can become coaches? I then describe a model of best practice that has helped shape the coaching approach described here. Next, I briefly discuss prior approaches to coaching that were foundational to my own work, followed by a description of the dynamic coaching approach. Critical features, or tenets, of this coaching approach are based on the evidence from best learning and instructional practices and on the evidence from the motivational interviewing (MI) approach. This chapter is focused on the structure and dynamic processes of coaching that reinforce self-regulation. Here I provide an overarching framework while describing the process of coaching, with practical forms and checklists to be used by coaches and students together to help guide the instruction in self-regulation. The examples of how to use these documents when coaching self-management, self-learning and studying, and self-advocacy are provided in Chapters 6 and 7. Thus, in this chapter I explain how coaches can best foster, support, and instruct college students in self-regulation.

WHO ARE DYNAMIC COACHES?

Professionals who have experience working with older adolescents and adults with executive function problems can learn to use a dynamic coaching approach. The scope of practice of educators, speech–language pathologists, occupational thera- pists, psychologists (vocational, rehabilitation, educational), neuropsychologists, and vocational rehabilitation professionals includes some of the basic knowledge and skills needed to work with these students. Being certified and/or licensed to practice in your state is the most basic requirement. However, additional knowl- edge and skills are typically necessary to fill in gaps in professionals' training to work with specific, selective groups of individuals. For example, an educator who has experience working with adolescents with developmental challenges would need additional training to be able to coach college students with acquired disabilities, such as TBI (including concussion), stroke, and other diseases of the brain. Likewise, a rehabilitation professional who is experienced in medical mod- els of practice may have the knowledge and skills to work with individuals with acquired brain injury, but have little understanding of the challenges faced by col- lege students with developmental disabilities and, thus, be in need of further edu- cation. Regardless of one's training, most professionals who work with college stu- dents with disabilities have not been trained to coach. Educators are accustomed to working with didactic instructional models, and rehabilitation professionals with medical treatment approaches. However, for both professions, research evidence now demonstrates that instructional practices such as direct instruction and meta- cognitive strategy instruction provide optimal results for training individuals to use specific strategies (Ehlhardt et al., 2008; Kennedy et al., 2008; Swanson, 1999; Tate et al., 2014).

MODELS FOR COACHING STUDENTS IN EXECUTIVE FUNCTIONS

There is no doubt that most behavioral models of coaching include the important work of Prochaska's stages of change. Take the example of the student who, no mat- ter how much he discussed the problem situation and no matter how many strate- gies and solutions he said he would try, he did not follow through. At each session, the student had all kinds of reasons for not acting on the plan, which involved study strategies to help him get an A in the class. The stages of change allow coaches to view student behavior along a continuum, which ranges from precontemplation to maintenance (DiClemente & Velasquez, 2002; Prochaska, DiClemente, & Norcross, 1992). Originally intended to help individuals who were trying to change addictive behaviors, these stages of changes have now been used to explain and facilitate changes in complex yet routinized behaviors. The five stages of change are listed in Table 4.1, along with useful strategies for coaches that can help facilitate movement to the next stage. The student in the example presented here appears to be recycling through the *planning* stage at coaching sessions, but is unable to put any of these strategies into *action*. A coach, using the strategies shown in the table, would revisit the student's commitment to reaching his goal, as well as the costs and benefits of using these strategies typically at the *contemplation* stage. The result might be that the student revealed that he was reluctant to implement study strategies because doing so would be too time-consuming and take time away from participating in an important campus organization that was directly related to his chosen career, a high priority for him. Thus, a coach would conclude that the costs and benefits had not been realistically and explicitly explored with the student. Once this was done, the student could decide to readjust his original goal of getting an A to getting a B in the class and to use study strategies that he had used in the past. Since these strategies were already familiar, they required less effort and time and could be implemented with ease. Note that students can get stuck at different points in the process, and knowing how to discuss this problem and instruct the student about ways to move past it depends on having a trusting relationship with the student, giving the student autonomy, fostering open communication, and validating that these kinds of decisions are complicated.

In 1998, Ylvisaker and Feeney were the first to describe a *collaborative approach* between rehabilitation clinicians and clients with ABI. In this approach, clinicians create hypotheses, which they systematically test while partnering with clients. *Problem solving* and *reciprocal adjusting* between the clinician and client are used until positive behavioral routines were solidified. Later, Ylvisaker (2006) described a self-coaching approach that was specific to the *contexts* in which the behavior occurred. Contexts are natural environments, including home, work, and school, where clients receive regular feedback from individuals they encounter naturally, and not just clinicians.

Quinn, Ratey, and Maitland (2000) described coaching pertinent to college students with ADHD. Like Ylvisaker and Feeney (1998), these authors emphasized *the relationship* between coaches and students as one "that merges the potential for growth of the individual with the skills of the coach" (p. 11). The coach helps and supports an individual in achieving personal goals while providing him or her with structure, supervision, and feedback. Practical examples of coaching students with ADHD were provided in daily living, academic, personal, and social skills.

TABLE 4.1. Stages of Change and Complementary Coaching Strategies for Students with Executive Function Problems

Stages of change	Description and example	Suggested coaching strategies
Precontemplation	*Description:* This is the earliest stage, where the person is unaware of the problem. He or she resists, rebels, resigns, or rationalizes, and does not acknowledge that a problem exists. *Example:* The student denies having memory and organization problems that resulted in missing assignments and poor test grades.	Depending on whether the student resists, rebels, resigns, or rationalizes: • Acknowledge that change is hard. • Listen to the reluctant student and be empathetic. • Embrace their independence while offering options, choices. • Build confidence by identifying strengths that can be used to compensate for weaknesses. • Have the student identify the pros and cons of his or her current behavior or situation. Summarize the balance without using cons as ammunition.
Contemplation	*Description:* The person acknowledges that there is a problem, but does not necessarily see the cause of or the solution to the problem, although he or she investigates potential solutions. The person may ruminate, weighing pluses and minuses over and over again. *Example:* The student realizes that his or her poor organization and memory problems have resulted in missing assignments and poor test grades.	• Listen carefully and empathetically. • Provide educational information that is personalized to the student's abilities/ disabilities. • Provide feedback so that the student can see/weigh consequences. • Find out how long the student has been aware of the problem and has been ruminating. • With the student, make pros and cons explicit, tipping the balance in the direction of change. • Affirm that the student can change.
Preparation	*Description:* The person is ready for change. He or she may have tried but failed in the past to change and needs to make plans for and a commitment to change. *Example:* The student creates a study plan and selects study strategies. The plan may be elaborate or simple.	• Actively listen to the student's ideas about plans, solutions, and strategies. • Assess how strong the commitment to change really is. • Support the student to make realistic, specific plans; vague plans may mean no plans. • Provide choices/options in plans, solutions, and strategies. • Introduce the idea that some plans, solutions, and strategies are ones that can be used in other situations. • Gently warn against recycling plans that failed in the past. • Use personal experiences with plans as examples of what did and what did not work.

(continued)

TABLE 4.1. *(continued)*

Stages of change	Description and example	Suggested coaching strategies
Action	*Description:* The person puts the plan into action, which involves changing one's behavior. Note that putting plans into action does not always equate with reaching a goal. *Example:* The student implements the study plan and study strategies. This can include modifying the action plan to fit the situation.	• Affirm the student's success at putting the plan into action. • Provide ways for the student to track the use of the plans/strategies and to track whether or not the plan is working (i.e., the goal is being realized). • Discuss modifications to the goal and/or plan based on the student's and others' feedback. • Relate action steps back to the self-regulation process.
Maintenance	*Description:* The person maintains the desired behavior using the plan, though relapse and recycling through the stages again is possible. *Example:* The student continues to implement the plan. He or she may discontinue its use if the routine was not well established or if something interrupts the routine and the student recycles to a prior stage to get started again.	• Acknowledge that maintaining a new plan or routine is challenging; it's hard work. • Support the student when he or she relapses into old study habits, time management routines, and ways of coping to encourage persistence and resiliency. • Use examples of exercise routines or diets to explore why people do not maintain new routines. • Create a plan with the student to resume the plan, or create a new one if the old no longer applies.

Note. Synthesized from DiClemente and Velasquez (2002) and Prochaska, DiClemente, and Norcross (1992).

Problem-based learning is another fundamental element of many coaching approaches. Here students learn to identify problems, create goals, develop plans while considering potential barriers, and put their plans into action. Swartz, Prevatt, and Proctor (2005) described a problem-based learning approach in which graduate students coached other college students with ADHD. Finn, Getzel, and McManus (2008) and Parker and Boutelle (2009) described a similar approach, which is used at Landmark College, a college for students with learning differences and disabilities.

Coaches use specific types of questions that model reflective thinking and prompt students' ability to plan and carry out their goals. By relying on questions as a primary tool for communication . . . coaching [focuses] on a student's capacity to take action on life goals. Coaches view students as creative and resourceful while helping them learn how to take action to accomplish goals that are important to them. (Parker & Boutelle, 2009, p. 205)

Indeed, Landmark College's Coaching Services Mission Statement states:

Through a process of inquiry, coaching offers support, structure, strategies, and guided practice that encourage students to understand and value themselves as they learn to take actions toward the realization of their goals. Students are seen by the coach as creative and resourceful and thus, with increasing self-awareness, as fully capable of discovering their own answers. (Parker & Boutelle, 2009, p. 206)

A DYNAMIC APPROACH TO COACHING SELF-REGULATION

Our model of coaching integrates many aspects of the approaches just described but also includes dynamic and self-regulation components. This model is based on not only the scientific evidence (e.g., Ben-Eliyahu & Bernacki, 2015) but also on our practical experiences coaching college students with brain injury (Kennedy & Coelho, 2005; Kennedy & Krause, 2011; Kennedy, Krause, & O'Brien, 2014).

So what is dynamic coaching? Dynamic coaching is an approach that supports and instructs individuals in the use of their own executive functions to be able to assess situations accurately and to solve problems that arise in order to accomplish both their proximal (immediate) and distal (long-range) goals. The term "dynamic" is used here because self-regulation processes are ongoing and ever changing, just as are students' academic needs and the contexts in which they find themselves. As Parker and Boutelle (2009) summarize, "Reports of clinical practice suggest that didactic models [of instruction] may not hold great efficacy for students who can quickly learn effective study skills but experience chronic difficulty employing those skills in a self-regulated manner" (p. 205). In other words, students with executive function problems can learn study strategies, but they struggle to implement them at a given time, for a given activity, and in an organized manner that makes sense in a particular context.

The critical features of our coaching approach are organized into four primary tenets. Here we have combined best practices for working with college students with disabilities with best practices in cognitive rehabilitation therapy into what we call "dynamic coaching."

- *Tenet 1.* Dynamic coaching is built on a trusting relationship between the coach and the student.
- *Tenet 2.* The structure of dynamic coaching both models and facilitates self-regulation.
- *Tenet 3.* Dynamic coaching occurs within the context of college where natural learning takes place and where outcomes are practical, functional, and student-centered.
- *Tenet 4.* Dynamic coaching explicitly instructs self-regulation as a way of thinking, doing, and reflecting.

Tenet 1. Building Relationships through Dynamic Coaching

The ultimate reason for using dynamic coaching with college students with executive function problems is to enable students to become the experts in how they think, learn, stay organized, and socialize in situations and during activities that are bound to change. One thing we know for sure is that college students will continue to develop and adjust as they face challenges in college that are similar to the challenges that they will face long after they graduate. And because these students are changing, the goals for which they are striving are bound to change as well. How do professionals from education, vocational rehabilitation, occupational therapy, and psychology, and speech–language pathologists and disability specialists, who are used to being the experts, provide support and facilitate change in college students whose disabilities lie in the very mechanisms that help them to navigate college independently, so that they become their own experts? *We can do this by building collaborative relationships with students and by explicitly instructing them about how to self-regulate in a variety of academic settings and for a variety of purposes.*

With an eye toward the goal of students' becoming their own experts, coaches motivate, inspire, model, instruct, support, and guide. But how will coaches accomplish this so that eventually there is a shift from the "coach as expert" to the "student as expert" within the college context? Coach–student partnerships must be formed to make this transition (Parker & Boutelle, 2009; Quinn et al., 2000; Ylivsaker, 2006; Ylivsaker & Feeney, 2009). These partnerships are created through mutual respect and the belief that students with disabilities hold *valuable, idiosyncratic knowledge about themselves* based on their past experiences and, to some extent, on their present experiences as a college student. How these ideas get communicated to college students with executive function problems is critical. MI techniques offer coaches practical ways of communicating that reinforce the message that at first students and coaches will figure out these challenges together, and then eventually, that students themselves will find solutions to their challenges. As one college student stated "Oh, I get it! I'll become my own coach!" MI is a style of communication that is

> a collaborative, goal-oriented style of communication with particular attention to the language of change. It is designed to strengthen personal motivation for and commitment to a specific goal by eliciting and exploring the person's own reasons for change within an atmosphere of acceptance and compassion. (Miller & Rollnick, 2013, p. 29)

There are four basic principles for coaches to follow: (1) express empathy, (2) develop discrepancy, (3) roll with resistance, and (4) support self-efficacy (Miller & Rollnick, 2002). MI was originally used by addiction counselors, but subsequent meta-analysis found significant and meaningful effects of using MI from randomized controlled trial studies targeting health changes in individuals with conditions such as diabetes, high blood pressure, and high cholesterol (Lundahl, Kunz, Brownell, Tollefson, & Burke, 2010; Rubak, Sandbaek, Lauritzen, & Christensen, 2005). Furthermore, a recent meta-analysis showed that when professionals used MI communication skills, clients were more likely to use language representative of change and less likely to use language representative of not changing (Magill et al., 2014).

The use of MI communicates mutual respect and the belief that students are autonomous through the key elements of active listening and questioning. Miller and Rollnick (2002) explain that a professional uses questions and responses that elicit change by

> (1) asking *open* questions that pull for change talk; (2) *affirming* and reinforcing the client for change talk; (3) *reflecting* back, sometimes selectively, change talk that the client has voiced, which allows him or her to hear it a second time; and (4) offering collecting, linking, and transitional *summaries* of change talk, allowing the client to hear once again the statements that he or she has made. (p. 83)

This MI approach, called OARS (asking Open questions, Affirming, Reflecting, and Summarizing), can be used by coaches to guide students in conversations about change (see examples in Chapters 5, 6, and 7). Table 4.2 has brief definitions of these kinds of questions and examples that could be used when coaching students through complex situations.

Strong conceptual and scientific evidence favors not only using MI with college students with substance abuse problems, but also with individuals with ADHD, learning disabilities, and brain injury. Two separate reviews of MI interventions used with college students with problem drinking were collectively found to reduce alcohol consumption and problem drinking (Branscum & Sharma, 2010; LaBrie, Cail, Pedersen, & Migliuri, 2011). When MI was added to each of two interventions for adolescents with ADHD, planning and solution-focused treatments, significant improvement was found and maintained at 3 months after the end of treatment (Boyer, Geurts, Prins, & Van der Oord, 2014). Furthermore, improvement was found in neuropsychological test results, parental reports of planning problems and executive functions, comorbid symptoms, and teacher reports. The results from this large (N = 159) randomized controlled treatment trial are in contrast to generally poor outcomes from other kinds of intervention for adolescents with ADHD.

MI is also effective when working with individuals with ABI (e.g., Bomdardier & Rimmele, 1999). Hsieh, Ponsford, Wong, and McKay (2012) found that MI techniques delivered *before* cognitive-behavioral therapy resulted in less anxiety and less nonproductive coping in adults with TBI who suffered from anxiety. For

TABLE 4.2. MI Questions (OARS) and Examples That Could Be Used When Coaching Students Through Complex Situations

Type of questions and statements	Shows that the coach . . .	Examples
Open questions (O): Questions that encourage rich and complex responses rather than simple either/or responses.	Is sincerely interested in understanding and empathizing.	• "Tell me about how it went on your first day at your new job." • "Tell me what you've noticed when you get really tired." • "Tell me more."
Affirmations (A): Statements that positively communicate your understanding without judgment.	Acknowledges the student's feelings, desires, goals, dreams, ideas, etc.	• "You've really put a lot of thought into this." • "It sounds like there are some reasons for not using your accommodations."
Reflections (R): Statements that reflect empathy and promote a deep level of understanding.	Is aware of the complexity of the situation, even its pros and cons, while moving the student toward change.	• "I understand how challenging this must be for you. It's not easy and there are lots of things to consider."
Summaries (S): Statements that synthesize what you've heard and what you understand.	Understands the situation by creating a brief synopsis. Provides an opportunity for clarification so as to avoid misinterpretation by the coach or the student.	• "OK, so tell me if I understand this correctly. You can go to disability services to take exams in the distraction-free room, but it sounds like it's too much trouble or hassle for you."

Note. Synthesized from Miller and Rollnick (2002, 2013) and MacFarland (2012).

a review of how MI applies to the recovery and rehabilitation of individuals with brain injury, readers are referred to Medley and Powell (2010), and for how MI applies to working with individuals with communication disorders, readers are referred to McFarlane (2012).

Besides using MI to establish partnerships, coaches can also *explicitly* communicate to students that they are the experts in all kinds of important information about themselves: how they think, what they like, what they dislike, how they feel, what motivates them, how they relate to others, strategies that have worked (or not worked) in the past, and their short-term goals and long-term plans, for example. Students have a "sense of self" that needs to be shared with coaches, which can be facilitated by the trusting and supportive relationship made possible by MI. MI implicitly reinforces this partnership, but it is critically important to explicitly tell students that they are also experts. Form 4.1 illustrates how a coach could explain this dynamic approach to students and others.[*] Additional resources on MI include publications by Berger and Villaume (2013), Miller and Moyers (2006), and Rosengren (2009).

---

[*] All reproducible forms are at the ends of chapters.

Besides coaches, students need other people to provide them with support as well. Students who have family and friends and other professional supports are more likely to be resilient and persistent when faced with academic, social, and emotional disappointments (Wyman, Cowen, Work, & Parker, 1991). Thus, students are encouraged to *form a team* of individuals who are aware of their disabilities and are trustworthy. The process by which students decide who should be on their team and what role team members will play is discussed in detail in Chapter 7.

Finally, coaches must be aware and respectful of how students cope in new and/or stressful situations. Some college students are very open to trying out new approaches if they think they will prevent a problem from happening. These "problem-focused," also called "solution-based," students are planners who tend to be actively engaged and embrace preventive measures (Krpan, Stuss, & Anderson, 2011a, 2011b; Lazarus & Folkman, 1984). Students can also be planners, but have a wait-and-see approach to new situations. These students tend to be more comfortable with trial-and-error learning that involves relying on old strategies or routines. They learn from their mistakes. The key here is that they learn, even though it's on an "as-needed" basis. However, some students tend to avoid situations in which they have experienced or anticipate experiencing stress. Students with this kind of emotion-based, avoidant coping tend to have lower overall outcomes after brain injury (Anson & Ponsford, 2006; Dawson, Cantanzaro, Firestone, Schwartz, & Stuss, 2006). Students with avoidant coping styles may get stuck at times and be unable to advance toward reaching their goals; these students in particular need the skills of a coach who guides and instructs them in more active planning using a supportive and accepting MI approach and self-regulation instruction. Table 4.3 includes a list of dos and don'ts of good coaches, who use MI to dynamically instruct and support these students as they learn to self-regulate while attending college.

Tenet 2. Structuring Dynamic Coaching to Model and Facilitate Self-Regulation

There are four phases to dynamic coaching, which are in themselves a framework that models self-regulation. These phases are represented in Figure 4.1 on page 68 and explained in detail in the remaining chapters in this book. In many ways, these phases are similar to Sohlberg and Turkstra's (2011) Planning, Implementation, and Evaluation (PIE), an organizational framework for professionals to follow while providing cognitive rehabilitation to individuals with brain injury. For our purposes, PIE is a framework by which professionals are continually reevaluating their goals and intervention. In our application of PIE, coaches and students *partner together.*

TABLE 4.3. What Good Coaches Do and Do Not Do

What good coaches do	What good coaches do not do
Explicitly model self-regulation.	Assume that students will do this implicitly.
Acknowledge the complexity of situations.	Oversimplify the reality of situations.
Collaborate with students in weighing pros and cons.	One-sided instruction in which students are the "recipients."
Tell students that the best solutions require collaboration.	Create solutions without student's collaboration.
Model how goals, strategies, and plans change.	Give the impression that these goals, strategies, and plans are set in concrete.
Hold students accountable.	Come down harshly or ignore students' mistakes.
Know that they cannot solve all of a student's problems; they know when to refer.	Believe that they can "do it all" and act accordingly.
Ask open, affirmation, reflection, and summary questions.	Tell, lecture, or "strongly recommend."
Motivate.	Shame by using "should."
Encourage autonomy and a relationship of trust.	Encourage dependency.
Provide support when it is needed.	Provide support when it is not needed or requested.
Express sympathy and empathy.	Blame.
Believe in and respect students' desires and preferences.	Believe that students are not trustworthy.
Facilitate students' choices.	Tell students what to do without choices.
Show students how to self-advocate and seek help from others.	Encourage students to be completely self-sufficient.
Encourage discussions about mistakes, poor decisions, or "It's just not working."	Discourage discussion by moving too quickly in an attempt to "fix it."

In *information gathering and evaluating,* coaches and students gather and evaluate information that helps to identify student strengths, challenges, preferences, beliefs, and goals. Through the use of MI and of surveys and questionnaires, this phase is typically done in the first few coaching sessions as the coach and the student review clinical reports, transcripts, and accommodation requests. This phase also includes supplemental testing if deemed necessary and a semistructured interview based on student responses to questionnaires and surveys. This phase is described in detail in Chapter 5.

The second phase of coaching, *interpreting and planning,* is derived directly from the first phase. Here the coach and student interpret or translate the information they've gathered from reports, questionnaires, and interviews. This is a collaborative process in which the student begins to learn how to think about what he

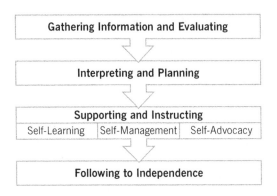

FIGURE 4.1. Phases of coaching.

or she is good at and where he or she is challenged, while the coach provides individualized education about how executive function problems relate to everyday academic and social activities. As they start collaborative planning, the coach and student identify immediate academic needs or proximal goals, and long-term, or more distal, goals. These plans also arise naturally from the discussions about students' abilities, preferences, and desires. This second coaching phase is described in Chapter 5 since it is integrally connected to gathering information and evaluating. Practical tools and forms are provided to guide this process.

The *support and instruction phase,* the third phase of coaching, involves explicitly instructing students in self-regulation. "How" one coaches self-regulation is critically important and is described later as tenet 4. Here, it is sufficient to state that once goals are identified, plans that include learning, practicing, and using new strategies are created, and ineffective strategies are eliminated. Thus, this phase of coaching is organized around three domains that are commonly identified as challenges to students with executive function problems: time management and organization; learning and studying (both of which are detailed in Chapter 6); and self-advocacy (discussed in Chapter 7).

The support and instruction phase of coaching also includes providing strategy options for students to select from that supports their autonomy in decision making. Some students, depending on their capability for learning new strategies, will need explicit and direct instruction to understand and use a new strategy. These individuals will need more intense rehabilitation that typically requires several instruction sessions a week that may continue for several weeks or even months. Most students who go to college though have sufficient memory and learning ability to learn new strategies fairly quickly. Sohlberg and Turkstra's (2011) book on optimizing cognitive rehabilitation is recommended for those who are unfamiliar with best practices in instruction since it is beyond the scope of this book to provide detailed steps to coaches in how to instruct.

Once strategies, plans, and solutions have been implemented, the student and coach reevaluate the usefulness of the strategies that the student implemented, which is typically based on student-provided documentation that is shared with coaches in their regularly scheduled sessions. At that time, students and coaches evaluate what happened, why it happened, and if adjustments need to be made to any of the goals, strategies, or plans. Thus, throughout coaching sessions, students experience what they are explicitly learning how to do: plan, implement, and evaluate (PIE). The situations college students with disabilities find themselves in forces the coach and the student to recognize a level of complexity and fluidity that requires constant reevaluation and adjustment.

The final phase of dynamic coaching typically involves mutually determining that students are becoming more adept at coaching themselves. This *independence and follow-up phase* typically takes place after a few semesters in which the coach has played less of an instructional role and more of a supportive one as students self-regulate. This phase can include administering tests, which may need to be done by coaches in professions in which testing is a requirement when billing for services. More important, however, are the use of surveys and interviews, self-reflection forms, and discussions of academic and vocational plans. These last two evaluation formats provide information about students' self-regulation, self-efficacy, and self-determination, since they reflect a student's gains toward independent thinking and problem solving. Self-reflection can be facilitated using two forms: one at the start of a semester or academic year (Form 4.2) and the other at the end of the semester or academic year (Form 4.3)

Maintaining contact with students in their remaining semesters has proven to be critically important for some, but not all, students. By meeting with students at the beginnings of the next few semesters, coaches can offer help if it is needed. Some students need support when reviewing their courseload and in deciding which strategies and proactive solutions they will use in the forthcoming semester. Chapter 8 describes the processes of following students as they become independent.

Besides the overarching phase structure of our coaching model, the schedule for coaching differs from both the intensive cognitive rehabilitation that individuals with ABI receive and from the sporadic tutoring sessions that students are familiar with. Weekly coaching sessions in the first semester forces college students with disabilities to be more accountable, unlike the more frequent outpatient rehabilitation appointment, in which as outpatients they can be more passive recipients of therapy, and unlike tutoring sessions where the content is narrowly defined and limited to a specific class. Attending coaching sessions with information about what went well, what did not go well, and what new challenges they anticipate, students are supported in how to reexamine and readjust their goals and/or the plans for achieving them. When students do not attend coaching sessions, they miss the opportunities to review and discuss the results of real-life practice; they are left to conclude "well, that just didn't work," or "using that strategy was too much work," or "it took too much time." If not required to, many students are not intrinsically motivated to try to figure out why the plan didn't work, and how and what to change the next time. Weekly coaching sessions create accountability; students become responsible for following through with "the plan" with the help of a coach. In the second or third semester, decreasing the frequency of these coaching sessions can occur after students take more responsibility in accomplishing their goals through planning, strategizing, and better follow-through.

Tenet 3. Context Creates Natural Learning and Outcomes

The college context in which coaching occurs is critically important in assessing outcomes. An athletic metaphor helps to explain this. Athletic coaches know that practicing skills outside of the game is needed when athletes are initially learning the fundamentals and specific skill sets. Demonstrating skills in drills comes first, and practicing skills in practice games is the next step. But nothing replaces the intensity and pace of the real game; there is a level of importance that cannot be matched in practice. Real games are full of tension, quick decision making, and changes based on what the opposing team is doing. The college experience is similar; it is dynamic, fluid, and complicated. The self-regulation that occurs in college is also dynamic, fluid, and complicated (Ben-Eliyahu & Bernacki, 2015). This is the context in which skills should be learned, in the context in which they will be useful and have many positive outcomes (Lichtinger & Kaplan, 2015).

Unfortunately, context is often excluded from best-practice models in medical rehabilitation and education. For example, the American Speech–Language–Hearing Association model includes "1) current scientific evidence including published systematic reviews, meta-analyses, randomized controlled trials, case reports and expert opinion; 2) clients' abilities, disabilities, goals and values; and 3) clinicians' expertise and decision-making skills" (*www.asha.org*). An obvious omission is the context. Fortunately, others have included context in models of best practice (Kennedy, 2014; McCauley & Fey, 2006). When coaching college students, the college context is critical for several reasons.

First, the context of college guides coaches toward recommending strategies that can be implemented quickly and from which the outcomes can be both immediately observed and have long-term impact. Clinicians trying to convince an outpatient with a brain injury to use a memory strategy often get met with resistance until that individual gets back to a college campus or a work setting where she or he understands the relevance of such a strategy, uses it while studying, and then observes the positive results on a quiz or exam. Individuals with brain injury may see little need for such strategies until they get experiential feedback from real academic and social activities, that indeed, strategies may help. But there is a long-lasting impact of having students meet their short-term goals, for example, improved grades results in many more positive opportunities such as being in a major of one's choosing. "Thus, the context has important functional relevance; the context provides reasons for using strategies by demonstrating the 'value added' [to the student]" (Kennedy, 2014, p. 284).

Second, a college campus is rich with real-life experiences that bring students with executive function disorders face-to-face with the realities of their disabilities. This will affect students' self-determination, or their sense of themselves, as they attempt some of the most challenging types of learning they have encountered. Negative and positive academic and social experiences will occur naturally, but a coach can provide a self-regulatory model and way of thinking about these experiences in a supportive manner, so that students can consider their options and begin to make changes.

Third, going to college provides an abundance of natural, timely, and rich experiences that require both quick, routine decisions and slow, more effortful decisions. Professions in medical, allied health, and education training programs have long known that there is only so much that one can learn by reading textbooks and attending class; that to really know how to apply what you learn, you have to use what you learn in natural situations where it is needed. In fact, there is a wealth of research findings on the effects of self-regulated learning and its relationship with problem-based learning among students in medical professions (e.g., Demiroren, Turan, & Oztuna, 2016; Loyens, Magda, & Rikers, 2008). Thus, students are placed in real-life practical situations where they must use self-regulation to create goals and plans and apply solutions and strategies and then quickly find out if they were effective or not.

Fourth, context-based learning in a natural environment enhances learning of new information in ways that are supported by research evidence. Educational and cognitive psychologists maintain that if you want to remember something, it is best to recall it, and not just repeat it, from your own memory at a later time. Compared with simple rehearsing, wherein something is simply repeated over and over, if the information is recalled after time has passed (during which you do something else), your chances of recalling it correctly later again are increased tremendously. Sometimes called "spaced retrieval," an emphasis is placed on the ever-expanding amount of time between when you learned the material and when you recalled it (Brush & Camp, 1998; Schefft, Dulay, & Fargo, 2008; Velikonja et al., 2014). However, recalling and stating (or writing) what you have recalled is a critical feature here as well. The idea here is that when you generate the response yourself, you are more likely to recall it at a later time; this has been referred to as "self-generation" and the "generation effect" (Velikonja et al., 2014). Both of these learning and practice techniques require deeper processing, which in turn results in better recall later. Importantly, these techniques occur naturally in college in various contexts, whether in class discussions when recalling lecture and reading material, in small-group projects with peers, while taking quizzes and exams, or in discussions with instructors during office hours.

Learning can also be enhanced through the way practice is scheduled. It turns out that we are more likely to retain a new procedure if practice is distributed over time than if practice occurs repetitively or all at once; this is called "massed practice." During the acquisition phase of a new strategy, students may need some massed practice, particularly if it involves a new procedure. However, after this initial practice, those who allow some time to pass before practicing the procedure again are more likely to recall the procedure at a much later time (see Sohlberg, Ehlhardt, & Kennedy, 2005, for a review). There is overlap between how to practice (spaced and self-generated) described here and when to practice (massed and distributed over time), but the point we make is that being in *college is the context* where these learning principles occur naturally.

Finally, the college allows students to experience the evidence (i.e., outcomes) that their solutions and strategies were effective. Considered "practice-based evidence" (PBE) (Wambaugh, 2007), in which outcomes are systematically documented as the intervention unfolds, this kind of evidence is very useful when the intervention and the outcomes have been tailored or individualized to meet the needs of students. Dynamic coaching is a perfect example of the kind of situations where PBE should be used. The practicality of student-generated, individualized goals reflects students' desire to succeed in college and to enjoy campus life. This focus on multiple, practical, student-centered goals is not new to fields of education nor to clinicians who provide outpatient cognitive rehabilitation to individuals with brain injury. However, the timeliness of dynamic coaching that occurs while students are enrolled in college differs from these other approaches in that, out of necessity, some goals are immediate (i.e., proximal) and strategies need to be learned and implemented quickly. And because some of their goals are long term (i.e., distal), students need immediate instruction in how to break goals down into doable and measurable steps.

Tenet 4. Instructing Self-Regulation through Dynamic Coaching

How do coaches teach self-regulation? Coaches should make self-regulation processes explicit when instructing students with executive function problems. Self-regulation is modeled and facilitated in several ways of thinking, planning, and doing that eventually become routine, automatic, and second nature for college students *and* for coaches. The evidence in favor of explicitly instructing individuals in these kinds of processes comes not just from cognitive rehabilitation for individuals with brain injury, but also from education research on students with ADHD/ADD and learning disabilities. Several reviews, including a meta-analysis of the intervention (Kennedy et al., 2008) aimed at improving executive functions in adults with TBI, have concluded that using metacognitive strategy instruction is effective when the goals reflect functional, everyday activities (Cicerone et al., 2011; Haskins et al., 2012; Swanson & Hoskyn, 1998; Tate et al., 2014). Examples of these kinds of therapy include time-pressure management training (Winkens, Van Heugten, Wade, & Fasotti, 2009), goal-management training (Levine et al., 2000), and self-talk procedures (Cicerone & Wood, 1987), which are all considered meta-cognitive strategies, but are presented to clients in a step-by-step manner that typically includes some kind of self-monitoring and self-reflection during the task and at its completion. Sohlberg and colleagues (2005) provided a review of how educational research has shown the effectiveness of an instructional approach called direct instruction, which is very similar to metacognitive strategy instruction in its emphasis on a step-by-step approach. Thus, the critical features appear to be step-by-step instruction paired with metacognitive processes (self-monitoring, self-selection, self-reflection, etc.).

So, how do coaches instruct college students in self-regulation? Instructing students in self-regulation involves explicitly modeling and instructing them in a way of thinking that requires them to engage in self-evaluation (or self-monitoring), self-control decisions, implementation and self-tracking, and comparing/adjusting to bring the process full circle. We use an expanded version of the self-regulation feedback loop presented in Chapter 1, Figure 1.1 (Kennedy & Coelho, 2005), but with several additional and explicit steps. These steps reflect research on self-regulated learning, on metacognitive strategy instruction, and on our own clinical experiences about where students face barriers and get stuck in the self-regulation process. Finding out where those barriers are in the self-regulation process and how to overcome them is the job of the coach and the student.

Figure 4.2 is an extension of the self-regulation process through which dynamic coaching occurs; it includes *all* of the steps involved in self-regulating complex activities. As such, these steps are organized by the part of the self-regulation framework within which they fall, Goals–Strategies–Act–Adjust (GSAA). This framework helps to organize each of the steps that coaches can explore with students to help them determine which part of self-regulation with which the student is having trouble. Each part of the GSAA approach to instructing self-regulation is described below.

First and foremost, students need to be able to self-evaluate (based on prior experiences) or, if no experience exists (e.g., the student just returning to college after a brain injury or entering college with a developmental disability), predict how they think they will do on an assignment, in a particular class, in a social situation, or even in a given academic major. As explained in Chapter 1, if students

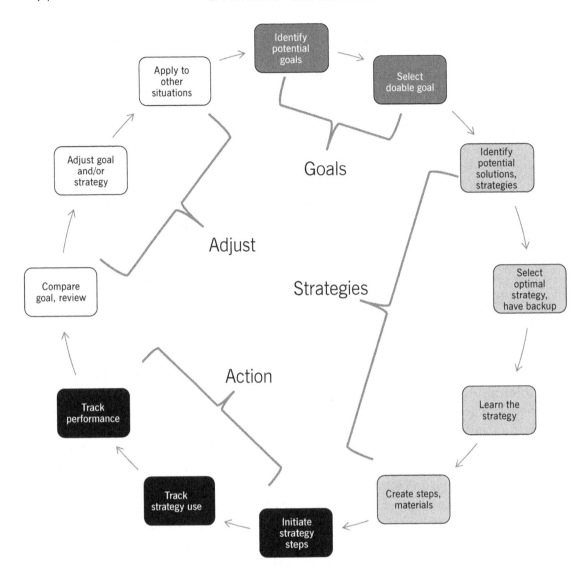

FIGURE 4.2. The self-regulation process in steps.

are not accurate at self-assessing, then they will not see a need for creating **goals** (as in <u>G</u>oals–<u>S</u>trategies–<u>A</u>ct–<u>A</u>djust), the first step in self-regulation. Thus, some level of self-assessment is a requirement for *creating goals,* and the first step in self-regulation coaching is to guide the student through a self-assessment discussion in the targeted area that is important to the student. Identifying possible goals, selecting doable goals, and making sure the goals are measurable is part of this process, and is discussed in more detail in Chapter 5.

Students may need more or less coaching assistance when first starting this process, depending on the degree to which they are self-aware of their abilities.

Self-awareness varies for different abilities and skill sets. For example, a student may be very aware of the challenges he experiences when trying to recall what he reads, but may be less aware of his tendency to monopolize a group conversation. Indeed, awareness of abilities that are tangible and observable, such as a physical disability, is more likely than being aware of thinking, learning, and conversational challenges both for students with and without ABI (e.g., Allen & Ruff, 1990; Giacino & Cicerone, 1998). Thus, a student may need little assistance when identifying learning or studying goals, but more assistance when establishing goals that involve communicating with peers and college personnel.

The next steps in self-regulation coaching involves *strategies and approaches to solutions* (as in Goals–Strategies–Act–Adjust) that will help these students achieve their goals. This involves selecting and learning to use strategies and making plans to implement their use. First, the coach and student discuss whether or not the student is using a strategy currently, and whether or not it has worked in the past and if it is likely to work now. This discussion centers on students' strengths and weaknesses; the information gained from professionals' evaluation reports (e.g., neuropsychologists, vocational rehabilitation professionals, and speech–language pathologists), surveys and questionnaires, and in-depth interviews are all done as a part of gathering information.

Of particular importance here are a coach's expertise and ability to identify evidence-based strategies that could be useful given the student's cognitive strengths and weaknesses and a coach's ability to use a metacognitive approach when instructing the student in the chosen strategy. When students are unfamiliar with specific strategies, coaches will need to instruct students in how to use them. Instruction is typically done within coaching sessions, where students can practice the new strategy initially with the coach, then practice it on their own. Chapter 6 details some studying and learning strategies that are effective for college students with memory and learning disabilities.

Equally important here is the coach–student relationship that encourages both of them to be involved with identifying potential solutions, but allows students to honestly report the likelihood of using a strategy; many well-meaning clinicians have taught students strategies or solutions, only to find out later that students did not follow through with using them. This collaborative relationship increases the likelihood that strategies and solutions will be ones acceptable to the student and that they will be implemented as planned. When students are actively involved in deciding and creating their own goals, they are more likely to be motivated to identify solutions and strategies and to practice the strategies and develop plans for implementing them.

The *"act"* (as in Goals–Strategies–Act–Adjust), the implementation phase of self-regulation, is critically important and is often overlooked or downplayed by those providing rehabilitation services. It is our experience that the action phase is a true test of both the strategy and of the collaborative relationship between coaches and students. If students have been fully engaged in identifying the goal, creating the plan (and anticipating barriers), they are far more likely to implement the strategy plan. Until students implement the strategy, neither the coach nor the student *really knows if it's "going to work"* and what the barriers will be. As students experience strategies that work (or don't work), that information turns into knowledge that they now have about their own strengths and challenges and what they need to do to succeed. First an action plan needs to be created, which typically includes gathering materials and setting up reminders. For example, a student using a recording device for taking notes would need to be sufficiently organized to remember to charge the device and bring it to the class where he is going to use it. A friendly reminder/alert set up on his smartphone could serve as the prompt that morning to put the device in his backpack.

As the strategy is being used, monitoring or tracking the strategy use is also part of the action phase. Discussing how strategy use will be tracked is a way to communicate to the student that this is truly his or her responsibility. Coaches can provide options for ways to do this, but many students come up with their own way to keep track. Some students like to use tracking forms that the coach provides, whereas other students use any number of apps that allow one to keep track. Tracking should also include how effortful or effortless and time-consuming it was. Tracking, along with the identification of any barriers, then become important issues to discuss at subsequent coaching sessions. Form 4.4 is a form that students and coaches can use to facilitate the discussion around the use of strategies.

Thus, the last step of the "action" phase of self-regulation involves having students report the outcome of using the strategy (or plan) to the coach and evaluating whether using the strategy was worth the effort and time. Besides tracking the use of the strategy, students should bring in "evidence" that the goal was met, such as graded assignments, exams, and papers, and report on their study habits and time management, which can involve use of study strategies, prioritizing, and even self-advocacy.

Reporting on strategy use in real academic situations is an essential part of coaching self-regulation that cannot be skipped. Our experiences with these students is that they often give up or abandon strategies too soon, typically after using a strategy once but with a less-than-optimum outcome; when this happens, they really don't know if continued use would help them reach their goal or not. Having these frank discussions with students are made easier by a coaching relationship built on trust and autonomy. Most students do not know how much effort or work will be needed to use a strategy until they have tried it. Coaches can reinforce the autonomy of students who identify barriers to using strategies by having a discussion about ways to deal with the barriers and trying to use the strategy again or about identifying other strategies that could avoid those barriers. The coach could reflect and summarize a discussion about options after hearing about the barriers:

STUDENT: I tried to use the smartpen for recording and taking notes in history. The desks are really small, and I had my backpack and latte to juggle. The instructor started before I could get everything set up right. That kinda threw me off to a bad start. I missed probably a good 10 minutes of important stuff.

COACH: So, it sounds like there were some issues around using this in class. Let's take a minute and chat about the barriers, and then you can decide if you want to try using the smartpen again and what needs to change to do that, OK?

Form 4.5 can be used to guide this conversation, with the student and coach listing the options together. The purpose of this exchange is to figure out what, if anything, needs to be *adjusted* (as in Goals–Strategies–Act–<u>Adjust</u>) by discussing (1) whether or not the goal or the strategy needs to change and (2) what that adjustment should be. Thus, the student will choose what he or she will do next. Our experiences are that often students can *easily decide what they want*, but have more difficulty *figuring out how* to get what they want. In guided conversations students are typically forthcoming in admitting whether or not they implemented the plan and whether or not the plan needs to be adjusted to something that is more realistic. If they return to the next coaching session without having implemented the plan, then coaches can help them identify the barriers that prevented them from implementing the plan, keeping in mind that these barriers can be environmental, attitudinal, social, or cognitive.

To accomplish some goals, such as large class projects, students may not need to learn or use new strategies. Rather, they may need to create a step-by-step plan to complete the project. Form 4.6 can be used to list each step and to have students predict if the steps will be easy, routine, or hard to complete. Self-regulation questions are provided to ensure that coaches and students explicitly discuss how well the plan (and its steps) was executed, making the processes of self-regulation explicit for students and coaches.

Some students may need additional conversations about not only how well a strategy worked, but also how much effort was involved in its use as compared to how helpful the strategy was, how important the goal really is, and, overall, if it is worth expending the effort. Form 4.7, Student Summary of Strategies, can be used by coaches to elicit tangible and explicit input from students when they find that a strategy is especially challenging to implement. Form 4.7 may be used in conjunction with Form 4.5, Strategy Usefulness and Next Steps, as coaches and students discuss the reality of using particular strategies.

When a strategy results in students achieving their goals, then the final part of self-regulation involves using this same strategy in different activities, for different goals, and under different conditions. Generalization or transfer of skills to untrained activities is a traditional problem in nearly all areas of teaching and rehabilitation. Students with executive function disorders are at a unique disadvantage though, since the very abilities that are needed to apply strategies to untrained skills are the ones impaired. Therefore, coaches can encourage students to explicitly consider when and how these newly learned strategies could be used elsewhere. For example, the use of reminders (visual, auditory, electronic, or paper) for bringing what one needs to college classes could also be used to remind students what they need to bring to work, to social events, and to study sessions. Many students themselves can identify when, where, and how a particular strategy could be used, but initiating this explicit conversation is typically the responsibility of the coach. Form 4.8 enables the coach and student to discuss the strategy and its other uses explicitly. And because students will learn to use a wide variety of strategies over the course of several semesters, coaches should encourage them to create a portfolio of strategies, plans, solutions, and adjustments.

So there are clear differences between dynamic coaching and other forms of supporting and instructing college students. Table 4.4 summarizes the key aspects of the four tenets by contrasting this approach with didactic instructional approaches.

TABLE 4.4. Similarities and Differences between Dynamic Coaching and Didactic Instruction

Dynamic coaching	Didactic instruction
Coach provides individualized education.	Coach provides individualized education.
Both coach and student are experts.	Coach is the expert.
Emphasizes process and results.	Emphasizes process and results.
Coach asks questions; students select strategies.	Coach identifies and selects strategies.
Coach relies on interviews, questionnaires, and behavior to gather information about students.	Coach relies on test scores and behavior to gather information about students.
Coach models self-regulation and provides structure; students provide content.	Coach models, provides structure, and provides content.
Goals are identified by students with coaching guidance.	Goals are often independent of the instruction.
Occurs in context, in real time (e.g., on a college campus).	Occurs out of context (e.g., in the therapy room).
Team based; students select team members.	One-on-one therapy or instruction are typical.
Less intensive (e.g., one session per week).	More intensive (e.g., two to three times per week).
Process-based goals are as important as the product-based goals.	Product-based goals are important.
Distributed practice occurs naturally.	Practice is artificial, out of the context from which strategies will be used.
Feedback comes naturally, from multiple sources.	Feedback comes from the coach.
Self-regulation is emphasized (i.e., monitoring, implementing, adjusting).	Learning the strategy is emphasized.

STUDENT BENEFITS ASSOCIATED WITH COACHING

There are numerous benefits for students who learn to self-coach, and evidence for this comes from research in several disciplines, including coaching college students with brain injury, ADHD, and learning disabilities. The most obvious benefit is that students experience the tangible rewards of reaching their proximal academic and college goals, such as getting a B on a quiz, trying out for the college chorus, or speaking up more in class. Our experience with students with brain injury is that when they implement and explicitly practice a studying, writing, or reading strategy in context, they achieve their goal rather quickly (Kennedy & Krause, 2011). The same kinds of academic results are found in studies that have documented outcomes of coaching students with ADHD and learning disabilities as well (Parker & Boutelle, 2009; Parker, Field, Hoffman, Sawilowsky, & Rolands, 2011; Swanson & Deshler, 2003). These are not the only benefits students report from being coached.

Students who have been coached also report improved self-regulation skills. In a large cohort study of students with ADHD and/or learning disabilities, Zwart and Kallemeyn (2001) found that students reported being more motivated and more goal-oriented and had less anxiety on a self-regulation questionnaire, the Learning and Study Strategies Inventory—2nd Edition (LASSI). In mixed methods studies in which questionnaires and interviews are included as outcome measures, students with ADHD and/or learning disabilities (Parker & Boutelle, 2009) reported better time management and a better sense of setting and reaching their academic goals. In 2013, a randomized controlled trial was conducted on the effectiveness of coaching college students with ADHD (Field, Parker, Sawilowsky, & Rolands, 2013). One-hundred and sixty undergraduates from 10 colleges were recruited and randomly assigned to either a coaching or a comparison group. Trained coaches provided 6 months of coaching, and pre- and post-scores on the LASSI and the College Well-Being Scale (Field, Parker, Sawilowsky, & Rolands, 2010) were collected, as well as qualitative interviews. After 6 months, students who were coached had higher scores on the LASSI, including the self-regulation cluster. Furthermore, students who were coached scored higher than students who were not coached. Qualitative analysis of interviews had corroborated these findings (Parker et al., 2011). Students who were coached reported (1) a stronger sense of self-determination as they set and achieved goals; (2) improved time management skills; (3) more productive coping strategies; (4) more self-awareness and self-acceptance; (5) more accountability; and (6) more confidence, more empowerment, and less stress.

In adults with acquired brain injury, research has also shown improvements in self-regulation, including strategy use from coaching and similar experiential learning approaches. Toglia, Johnston, Goverover, and Dain (2010) reported that when adults with brain injury were explicitly instructed to use strategies across several different contexts, the self-regulation of strategy use changed positively, whereas overall self-awareness did not. Intervention consisted of only nine sessions though, which may account for the lack of change in self-awareness. In our 2011 study of two college students with TBI who were coached for two semesters, the students reported using more study strategies, learned time management skills, and made good decisions about balancing work, socializing, and college life (Kennedy & Krause, 2011). Furthermore, both students graduated in a major that they decided on while being coached and became employed in their chosen field. O'Brien, Schellinger, and Kennedy (2017) also found that, after being coached, college students with brain injury reported using a wider variety of solutions and strategies when questioned about time management and organization, studying and learning, and social situations.

A discussion of the benefits of using a coaching approach with college students would be incomplete without a discussion about resiliency and persistence. When the ongoing processes needed to self-regulate (i.e., self-monitoring, self-control, initiating action, comparing and adjusting) are considered, it becomes obvious that students with disabilities, especially those with dual disabilities that include executive function problems, need to be both persistent and resilient in order to succeed academically. Persistence is the ability to maintain an acceptable amount of effort and motivation to continue to engage in problem-solving processes in order to reach a goal. For example, the student who does not discuss the instructor's feedback on an assignment in which his grade was lower than he expected is not persisting toward the goal of getting a better grade next time, simply because he is unwilling to examine what went wrong. Instead, he employs an avoidance strategy by disengaging, and most likely will not reap the benefit of a deeper understanding of (1) the instructor's expectations and (2) how he might prepare differently for the next assignment.

The ability to "bounce back" can be seen in the ability to make changes in the strategy (e.g., seek help, use a different study technique, change the environment) or in the level of effort when the strategy did not work or the goal was not achieved. If students abandon or give up after an initial failed attempt, they will not have the opportunity to persist or to be resilient by making adjustments. The effects of being resilient and persistent are clear. College students who are resilient and persist are more likely to reach their academic goals (e.g., DeBaca, 2010; Herrero, 2014; Jowkar, Kojuri, Kohoulat, & Hayat, 2014); are less likely to experience anxiety, stress, and depression; and more likely to have positive self-determination (e.g., Kwok, Wong, & Lee, 2014). They have the awareness that if they fail, they will be able to figure out what went wrong and why and what could help next time. Brown (2010, p. 64), who researches hope and shame, summarizes the qualities that resilient people share, which applies to college students as well. In her view, resilient people:

1. Are resourceful and have good problem-solving skills.
2. Are more likely to seek help.
3. Hold the belief that they can do something that will help them manage their feelings and to cope.
4. Have social support available to them.
5. Are connected with others, such as family or friends.

These "bounce-back" qualities actually look very similar to our description of students who self-regulate and have a strong sense of self and self-determination. These are college students who take action by solving problems to achieve their goals, know where and how to get help when needed, have strong self-efficacy, and are connected to others who can provide them with support. Thus, *self-regulation and self-determination include the same skill sets that are present in individuals who are resilient!* And unlike characteristics that are immutable, like one's socioeconomic background, these are all dynamic processes that are fluid and can change.

It makes sense then that a by-product of coaching may be improved resiliency and persistence from the consistent support and instruction in self-regulation that students get from coaches and from the structure, accountability, and regularity of coaching sessions. And students with brain injury report that one of the benefits of having a coach was knowing that every week they had someone with whom they could discuss their challenges and achievements as they go through college while figuring out what they will do once they graduate. A group of experts who work with military populations views *resilience as a protective factor that promotes positive outcomes for service military and veterans* that enable these individuals to successfully return to the community and to college (Mashima et al., 2017, p. 8). They advise that clinicians and/or coaches can "cultivate" resilience by:

1. Focusing on recovery from setbacks rather than on failure or the problem itself.
2. Recruiting internal and external coping resources.
3. Anticipating challenges and preparing the [student] with compensatory strategies to minimize potential negative impact.
4. Highlighting optimism and hope when reinforcing mastery of goals.

In closing, Ylvisaker (2006) reminded us that indeed

the goal of self-coaching is to improve planful goal-oriented [behavior] and ultimately success . . . that self-coaching interventions also help the individual construct a positive image of self, associated with effective self-regulation/

self-coaching and ultimately successful social and vocational pursuits . . . self-coaching is ideally an everyday, context-sensitive intervention. (p. 248)

ADDITIONAL RESOURCES

- For coaching K–12 and older children with executive function problems, readers are referred to the book *Coaching Students with Executive Skill Deficits* by Dawson and Guare (2012).
- For coaching students who are on the autism spectrum, here is a sample of online resources:
  - *www.collegeautismspectrum.com/students.html*
  - *http://autismpdc.fpg.unc.edu/sites/autismpdc.fpg.unc.edu/files/imce/documents/NPDC_CoachingManual.pdf*
  - *www.iidc.indiana.edu/pages/Academic-Supports-for-College-Students-with-an-Autism-Spectrum-Disorder*
- For coaching students who have intellectual disabilities, here is a sample of online resources:
  - *www.thinkcollege.net*
  - *https://ici.umn.edu*
- For information on students with brain injury who are transitioning to college, see *http://cbirt.org.*
- For a description of Landmark College, a college specifically for students with different learning difficulties, see *www.landmark.edu.*

What to Expect with Dynamic Coaching

Dear _____ :

Dynamic coaching is a way to collaborate with an expert who knows how to support college students with executive function problems. Here are some ways in which this kind of coaching is similar to what an athletic coach does:

- Teaches skills that are necessary for college success.
- Provides support and feedback while you use these skills in college.
- Motivates you and keeps you on a path to meet your goals.
- Understands that using strategies in real life differs from just practicing them.

Because of your disability, you need a coach who knows and understands the unique challenges and adjustments that you face in college. Dynamic coaches are professionals who have the background and training to provide support and instruction while you attend college. These professionals can include speech–language pathologists, psychologists, occupational therapists, vocational rehabilitation counselors, educators, and disability specialists. They have expertise in working with students with executive function problems, and they will *partner with you to figure out what your strengths are, what your challenges are, and where and when you need support in college.*

This kind of coaching differs from athletic coaching, rehabilitation, teaching, and tutoring in several ways. In dynamic coaching:

- The goal is for "you" to become the expert in how you learn, manage your time, and make friends.
- You will learn to self-coach, that is, you will become your own coach.
- You will be a partner with your coach, so that together you will figure out what works, what doesn't, and how much time implementation takes.
- You will have autonomy in decision making during discussions with your coach.
- You will experience a highly individualized approach, based on your abilities, preferences, beliefs, and academic goals.

In this approach, students and coaches together identify goals and create solutions and strategies and implement them in three areas in which college students with executive function problems are challenged: (1) self-management and organization, (2) self-learning and studying, and (3) self-advocacy. These domains overlap considerably as part of college life, although the way in which they overlap is uniquely yours.

Your coach will take you through four phases of coaching: gathering information and evaluation, interpretation and planning, support and instruction, and independence and follow-up.

FORM 4.2

Self-Reflection: Start

Name: _____

Date: _____ Year and semester: _____

Number of courses and credits enrolled in this semester: _____

Instructions: Predict what your college experiences will be in the upcoming semester. Think about all aspects of your college life, including academic, social, work-related, daily living, and family experiences, that you will have. Fill in the blanks with as many examples as you can think of.

1. I think that _____ will be very challenging for me to handle this semester.

    _____   _____

    _____   _____

    _____   _____

    _____   _____

    _____   _____

    _____   _____

2. I think that _____ will be fairly routine for me to handle this semester.

    _____   _____

    _____   _____

    _____   _____

    _____   _____

    _____   _____

    _____   _____

3. I think that _____ will be easy for me to handle this semester.

    _____   _____

    _____   _____

    _____   _____

    _____   _____

    _____   _____

    _____   _____

Self-Reflection: End

Name: _____

Date: _____ Year and semester: _____

Number of courses taken and credits earned this past semester: _____

Instructions: Consider all of your experiences as a college student this past semester, including academic, social, work-related, daily living, and family experiences, that you have had. Fill in the blanks with as many examples as you can think of.

1. I have found that _____ was ABOUT AS challenging as I had expected.

_____   _____

_____   _____

_____   _____

_____   _____

_____   _____

_____   _____

2. I have found that _____ was MORE challenging than I had expected.

_____   _____

_____   _____

_____   _____

_____   _____

_____   _____

_____   _____

3. I have found that _____ was LESS challenging than I had expected.

_____   _____

_____   _____

_____   _____

_____   _____

_____   _____

Tracking **Strategy Action**

Instructions: Each day, rate your strategy use on the following scale: (0) not needed today; (1) not addressed; (2) attempted; (3) completed; (4) completed multiple times.

Strategy	Monday	Tuesday	Wednesday	Thursday	Friday	Saturday	Sunday	Notes

Strategy Usefulness and Next Steps

Instructions: This form can help you figure out what happened when you implemented the plan or strategy. You can also consider your options. Write out the strategy, describe what happened, consider your options, and identify what you want to do next.

Goal:

Strategy/plan:

Did you use it enough so you can tell if it worked?

Yes   No

Describe how well it worked:

✓ _____

✓ _____

✓ _____

✓ _____

Describe barriers that interfered:

✓ _____

✓ _____

✓ _____

✓ _____

What is your plan?

☐ Continue to use it as is and assess its usefulness.

☐ Continue to use it, but consider ways to make it easier and more effortless.

☐ Discontinue its use (and why) and select a different strategy.

☐ Discontinue its use, change your goal, and figure out the impact.

What is your plan?

☐ Do nothing different and try again.

☐ Deal with barriers and try again.

☐ Use a different strategy and, if so, what?

☐ Have a backup strategy if barriers return.

☐ Change your goal and figure out the impact.

Action-Planning Form

Instructions: Write out what you want to accomplish and the steps in your plan.

1. Anticipate how hard each step will be to get done.

2. When you are done, reflect back on the steps that you followed to see if they were about as difficult as you anticipated.

Goal:

Steps in my plan	Done (✓)	E = easy; R = routine; H = hard	
		Will be . . .	Was
1. Due date:			
2. Due date:			
3. Due date:			
4. Due date:			
5. Due date:			
6. Due date:			

(continued)

How well did this plan work? Did you accomplish your goal?

- Were all of the steps needed?

- Were there additional steps that you did not anticipate? Which ones?

- Were the steps as hard as you anticipated?

- Would you do anything differently next time?

Student Summary of Strategies

Strategy and Date	Importance	Use	Help	Effort	Worth
Briefly explain the strategy or plan What is it supposed to do? What's the goal?	How much do I care about achieving this goal?	How much or how often did I use the strategy?	How helpful was the strategy?	How much effort did this strategy take? How hard was it to use? 1 = a lot; 5 = very little	Was it worth it?
Rate responses as 1–5: (1) Not at all; (2) A little; (3) Somewhat; (4) Quite a bit; (5) Very much/All the time					

Strategy Review and Other Applications

Instructions: Consider the strategies you are now adding to your toolbox. List the strategies, and identify other situations or activities in which you could use them. SM, self-management; SL, self-learning; SA, self-advocacy.

Strategy	Domain: SM, SL, SA	Current use	Other uses

CHAPTER 5

Information Gathering and Collaborative Planning

Now that you have some foundational background about coaching from the previous chapters, we now turn to what coaches need to do first; that is, to evaluate students' strengths and weaknesses, find out students' preferences, identify their goals, and do so in collaborative ways that foster trust. Although MI is the dominant method for getting much of this information, other reports, surveys, and supplemental testing are typically needed to get a clear picture of students' abilities and disabilities.

The purpose of this chapter is not only to provide you with the tools (e.g., surveys, forms, checklists) that enable you to gather all of the necessary information; but importantly, its purpose is also to describe the coaching processes that will help students begin to discover their strengths and weaknesses, make plans and create goals, and implement and adjust those plans as needed. In other words, it is not enough to have forms or checklists for students and coaches to complete; coaches need to know how to use these forms to stimulate discussions that facilitate and support students in their own self-discovery. Therefore this chapter is divided into two broad sections:

1. Gathering information, with the following objectives:
   - To describe the information that needs to be collected and draw attention to tools that supplement more traditional tests.
   - To provide you with surveys and questionnaires that contain useful information about students' perspectives of their own executive functions.

- To describe how those tools are used to find out what strategies are being used and whether or not they are effective.
- To describe how the reports that document students' cognitive and executive function abilities can be interpreted for students' own understanding.

2. Collaborative planning, with the following objectives:

- To describe SMARTER (shared, monitored, accessible, relevant, transparent, evolving, and relationship-centered) goals and goal attainment scales.
- To describe the difference between performance goals and self-regulation goals and why this distinction is important.
- To describe how to create teams that provide support.
- To describe how coaches and students can plan for current and coming semesters.

QUESTIONNAIRES, INTERVIEWS, AND TESTS

A good coach gathers all of the necessary information to get a clear picture of the student he or she will be coaching. Answers to the following questions are needed so that the coach and student can get started.

- What is the origin of the student's executive function problems?
- What are the student's cognitive, academic, and social strengths and weaknesses?
- What are the student's other disabilities?
- What reasonable accommodations is the student currently receiving, if any? Is the student using his or her accommodations?
- What are the student's academic and vocational goals?
- What does the student perceive as the major barriers to reaching his or her goals?
- What does the student do for fun?
- Does the student have family and/or friends who are supportive?
- How does the student handle or cope with setbacks?
- What was the student's school experience growing up?

There are four ways to get answers to these kinds of questions.

1. The coach and student review important documents together (e.g., reports from clinical and educational testing, transcripts, accommodations documents).

2. The student is administered supplemental tests, if needed.

3. The student completes questionnaires and surveys.

4. The coach follows up the questionnaires and surveys with semistructured interviewing.

Figure 5.1 displays the components of this process and the sequence of steps that coaches go through to obtain all of the necessary information detailed in this chapter. Form 5.1 is a simple checklist to guide coaches as they get started, and Form 5.2 is a checklist sent to students *prior* to the first session and includes a list

Forms
- Demographic, Academic, Medical, and Social History Form (Form 5.3)
- Accommodations documentation from disability services
- Other forms (e.g., Form 4.1, What to Expect with Dynamic Coaching, Form 5.2, Getting Started Checklist for Students)

Reports
- Clinical reports of test results from various professionals
- Unofficial copy of transcripts
- List of currently enrolled courses
- Other relevant reports from professionals

Supplemental tests, surveys, and questionnaires (Table 5.1)
- Cognitive tests, including tests of executive functions
- Language tests, including tests of reading, writing, word-finding, vocabulary, etc.
- College Survey for Students with Other Disabilities (Form 5.4), College Survey for Students with Brain Injury (Form 5.5), and College Survey for Students with Concussion (Form 5.6)
- Learning style surveys
- Social and coping surveys
- Resiliency scales

Translating abilities and disabilities

Practical examples are listed and discussed with students (Form 5.8, Interpreting Abilities and Disabilities)

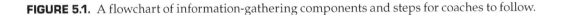

FIGURE 5.1. A flowchart of information-gathering components and steps for coaches to follow.

of documents that the students should provide during the first and/or second session. By requesting that students bring these documents to initial sessions, coaches can observe students' ability to be organized, to follow through with instructions, and to use strategies for getting documents that are not readily available.

First and foremost, coaches need a completed academic, medical, and social history from the student, as shown in Form 5.3. The form includes a set of questions for all students to answer, as well as questions specifically for students with brain injury (e.g., TBI/concussion, stroke, multiple sclerosis). Verifying the information on this form is a great way to start off the first coaching session, using the OARS question format from MI. This informal interview allows students to provide explanations and allows coaches to get more detailed information by using questions that begin to build a trusting relationship. Here are two examples of questions generated from information that a student provided on a history form.

Example of a Student with Brain Injury

COACH: I see that you have 23 college credits that you've completed and that you don't have a college major. [summary] Can you tell me more about those credits and what your thoughts are on a major? [open question]

STUDENT: Oh, they're mostly general education credits. I had wanted to major in history, thinking I'd go into law, and was trying to figure that out when I had my accident. I love history, always have . . . but now, after my brain injury, I just don't know if I'm going to be able to do all of that reading and writing . . . you have to have a good memory? So, yeah, I need to declare a major, but I need to figure out what I can actually do now, I mean, if majoring in history is realistic or not.

COACH: Well, you're certainly putting lots of thought into it, and you seem to know what could give you some trouble. [affirmation] I think we'll be able to figure out where your strengths are now and what you are going to need more help with too. [affirmation] When do you need to declare a major?

STUDENT: I'm not sure actually. I think it's when you're a sophomore. I need to check.

COACH: OK, so you've got some time before you have to do that. Is this a priority for you this semester?

STUDENT: Yeah, I just want to know so I can plan, but I don't really know where to begin. I don't want to take a bunch of classes that I won't need if I'm not going to be in that major.

COACH: All right, so this is really important and it affects your immediate decisions about what courses to take, which courses you may find difficult, and what you really want to do even after you graduate. [summary and reflection] Can I write this down and come back to it later when we are finished going through these documents? [permission]

STUDENT: Oh, sure.

Example of a Student with ADHD

COACH: So, you were diagnosed with ADHD once you were in college? [summary]

STUDENT: Yes, that's right. I always had problems controlling my attention growing up, and I was tested a few times. But each time the results were the same. I had some trouble with paying attention in class. Guess I was kinda impulsive. I'd get in trouble for doing things, but never bad enough to be in special ed or anything like that. And my grades were always good. My parents got me a tutor to help with trigonometry and calculus. Mostly I just figured it out on my own . . . doing things in class to make to help me pay attention and stay out of trouble.

COACH: Like what kinds of things did you do that helped? [open question]

STUDENT: Let's see . . . I would pretend I was somewhere else in my head, especially when the teacher was going on and on about something I could care less about. I would sit up really straight and stare at the teacher and nod, but be thinking about something else completely different.

COACH: And did that work? I mean, did it help you focus? And what if the topic was something you were really interested in? [open question]

STUDENT: If I'm interested, then I have no trouble paying attention. In fact, it's almost the opposite; sometimes it's hard for me to move on to do something different after that. It's kinda weird, you know? I'm sure there were better ways I could pay attention, but honestly that's what I did. Probably didn't help me remember stuff I didn't really care about, but it did keep me from getting in trouble.

COACH: Actually, it makes a lot of sense. [affirmation]

Supplemental Tests

Clinical reports from psychologists, neuropsychologists, speech–language pathologists, occupational therapists, vocational rehabilitation specialists, and other professionals can provide coaches with a comprehensive description of students' impairments, skills, and behavior, including but not limited to the following basic processes (from Table 1.1) and executive functions (from Table 1.2) in Chapter 1:

Basic Processes

- Cognition—attention abilities, visuospatial ability, alertness, memory retention, memory recall, memory recognition, visual and auditory sensations and perceptions.

- Language—word-finding, vocabulary, reading, writing, narrative skills, expository skills, reasoning, speed of processing, conversational and social skills.

- Emotions, psychological status—emotional status, anxiety, depression.

- Physical abilities—vision, hearing, mobility, writing, accessing technology, speaking ability, speed of movement, coordination.

Executive Functions

- Attention control—deciding what to pay attention to, and the ability to pay attention, to ignore, and to switch attention.

- Memory control—ability to use strategies to attend to and manipulate information in one's mind; ability to remember to do something later (i.e., prospective memory).

- Initiation—getting started and/or returning later to a course of action after stopping.

- Inhibition and impulse control—withholding urges to say and/or do at a particular time or place or in a particular circumstance.

- Problem identification and goal setting—identifying problems, setting goals, and planning activities to meet goals.

- Flexibility of thinking and behavior—switching and adapting viewpoints and ways of thinking.

- Emotional self-regulation—resiliency, coping strategies and behaviors, emotional self-management.

- Cognitive self-regulation—self-monitoring, selecting and using strategies, and making adjustments when given feedback.

The selection of supplemental evaluation tools depends on the information coaches are able to get from the already existing reports and how recently these tests were administered; if these tests were given more than a year ago, it is likely that some supplemental testing will be needed since we know that abilities and disabilities change as students recover from an injury or as they have more experience with college life.

While executive functions are often included in most clinical reports from psychologists, we have found that practical or functional evaluation tools are often missing, even though they provide some of the most useful information for both coaches and students. Table 5.1 lists examples of supplemental tests, surveys, and questionnaires that we have found useful in working with college students with executive function problems. Table 5.1 does not include tests that are part of large, standard cognitive and language batteries used to identify and document the type of impairments and the need for accommodations, such as the Delis–Kaplan Executive Function System (D-KEFS; Delis, Kaplan, & Kramer, 2001) and the Wechsler Adult Memory Scale–IV (Wechsler, 2009). A psychologist, speech–language pathologist, or occupational therapist usually administers these tests depending on the test publisher's criteria and requirements. The tests included in Table 5.1 measure performance that is closer to what students would demonstrate during functional activities (e.g., the Nelson–Denny Reading Test and the Functional Assessment of Verbal Reasoning and Executive Strategies [FAVRES]; MacDonald, 2005). The FAVRES has been found to be the best predictor of vocational status in individuals with brain injury (Meulenbroek & Turkstra, 2016). The only test listed in Table 5.1 that is not "functional" is the Repeatable Battery of Assessment of Neuropsychological Status (RBANS), which is a valid and reliable cognitive-impairment screening tool that takes 30 minutes to administer and can be administered by professionals other than psychologists . We use the RBANS when a more comprehensive battery of tests is missing. The tests listed in Table 5.1 are examples only and are not meant to be definitive.

Turkstra and colleagues (2005) reviewed standardized tests used by speech–language pathologists when evaluating the cognitive, communication, and language abilities of individuals with brain injury. Sixty-five tests were reviewed for their psychometric properties, including reliability and validity. The authors found that, while these tests provided information about the underlying processing impairments, they lacked information about the functional or everyday problems faced by individuals with TBI. These authors and others (e.g., Constantinidou & Kennedy, 2017; Wilson, 2003) have concluded that responses on surveys, questionnaires, and interviews and clinical observation better identify clients' and/or students' needs and help professionals create practical and functional goals.

Surveys, Questionnaires, and Interviews

Coaches need to know students' cognitive and language strengths and impairments from test results in order to understand the underlying processing deficits that are part of students' dual disabilities and to make informed strategy decisions to compensate for their deficits. Surveys and questionnaires provide a different kind of information; they are used to determine students' own perceptions of their abilities and disabilities, what strategies they are already using, and whether or not

TABLE 5.1. Surveys, Questionnaires, and Tests for Evaluating College Students with Executive Function Problems, Listed Alphabetically

Tools	Description
Behavior Rating Inventory of Executive Function—Adult Version (BRIEF-A; Roth et al., 2013)	A survey tool that captures everyday executive functions with self- and informant reporting. There are 75 items that encompass nine areas of executive function that have been found to correlate into two broad indexes: behavioral regulation and metacognition. Normed on adults from various diagnostic groups, including ADHD and TBI.
College Self-Efficacy Inventory (CSEI; Solberg, O'Brien, Villareal, Kennel, & Davis, 1993)	A survey tool of 20 items that capture level of confidence in completing academic activities. Course efficacy, roommate efficacy, and social efficacy emerged as three factors all related to self-efficacy.
College Students with Disabilities Campus Climate (CSDCC; Lombardi, Gerdes, & Murray, 2011)	A survey tool "designed to measure the impact of individual actions and perceptions on postsecondary and social supports on college students with disabilities" (p. 111). There are 43 items that aggregate around peer support, utilizing accommodations, disability services, self-advocacy, family support, faculty attempts to minimize barriers, and stigmatization.
College Survey for Students with Brain Injury (CSS-BI; Kennedy & Krause, 2009)	A multipurpose survey tool to capture perceptions of college students with brain injury. Injury history, associated symptoms, services received, and ratings of those services and life changes are included. Agreement ratings of 13 academic challenges clustered around time management and organization, studying and learning, psychosocial issues, and stress (Kennedy, Krause, & O'Brien, 2014).
College Survey for Students with Concussion and Other Injuries (CSS-CO; Kennedy, DeSalvio, & Nguyen, 2015)	Similar to the CSS-BI, this is a multipurpose survey tool to capture perceptions of college students with concussion. Injury history, associated symptoms, services received, and ratings of those services and life changes are included. Agreement ratings of academic challenges include judgments of time management, organization, studying and learning, and the impact of physical impairments on academic performance.
College Survey for Students with Other Disabilities (CSS-OD; Kennedy, 2016)	Similar to the CSS-BI and the CSS-CO, this survey tool is also multipurpose. Educational and medical history, associated symptoms, services received, and ratings of those services are included. Agreement ratings of academic challenges include judgments of attention needed for academic activities, time management, organization, and studying and learning.
College Well-Being Scale (CWBS; Field, Parker, Sawilowsky, & Rolands, 2010)	A 10-item assessment using a Likert-type scale that measures participants' perceptions of factors associated with well-being for students in postsecondary education.
Controlled Word Association Test (COWAT; Ruff, Light, Parker, & Levin, 1996)*	A subtest of the Multilingual Aphasia Examination (MAE) that assesses verbal fluency by evaluating the spontaneous production of words in a limited amount of time. The individual is provided with a letter (i.e., C, F, or L) and is given 1 minute to name as many words beginning with that letter. This is repeated for each of the three letters.

(continued)

TABLE 5.1. *(continued)*

Tools	Description
Functional Assessment of Verbal Reasoning and Executive Strategies (FAVRES; MacDonald, 2005)*	A test of reasoning and planning skills that has correlated with returning to work. There are four activities that require the use of cognition in everyday living situations. This standardized assessment identifies abilities in verbal reasoning, complex comprehension, discourse, and executive functioning in adults ages 18–79. It takes 60 minutes to administer this assessment.
Learning and Study Strategies Inventory (LASSI; Weinstein et al., 2002)	A 10-scale, 60-item standardized assessment tool designed to identify students' awareness, use of study strategies, and strengths and weaknesses related to skill, willingness, and self-regulation. The skill component targets information processing, selecting main ideas, and test strategies. The willingness component targets attitude, motivation, and anxiety. The self-regulation component targets concentration, time management, self-testing, and use of academic resources.
Mayo–Portland Adaptability Inventory (MPAI-IV; Malec, 2005)	A 35-item survey tool that identifies the current status of an individual with a postacute acquired brain injury. The three subscales (i.e., ability, adjustment, participation) represent the range of physical, cognitive, emotional, behavioral, and social problems that an individual may encounter.
Motivational Studying and Learning Questionnaire (MSLQ; Pintrich & DeGroot, 1990)	An 81-item self-report measure consisting of 15 subscales to assess college students' motivation to engage with course material and learning strategies. This test takes 20–30 minutes to administer.
Nelson–Denney Reading Test (Brown, Fishco, & Hanna, 1993)*	A reading test that includes both a vocabulary and reading comprehension/reading rate section for high school and college students and adults. The vocabulary test is a 15-minute timed test. The reading comprehension test is a 20-minute test, in which the first minute is used to determine the reading rate.
Repeatable Battery for Assessment of Neuropsychological Status (RBANS; Randolph, 2012)*	A screening test of cognitive impairments for adults with neurological involvement. Subtests screen immediate and delayed verbal and visual memory, attention, and category/word generation. It takes 30 minutes to administer and has two alternative forms.
Self-Regulation Skills Interview (SRSI; Ownsworth, McFarland, & Young, 2000)	A six-item tool used to measure emergent awareness, anticipatory awareness, readiness to change, strategy generation, degree of strategy use, and strategy effectiveness in those who sustained an ABI. These items identify the range of metacognitive skills necessary for rehabilitation planning, monitoring of an individual's progress, and evaluating the outcome of treatment interventions. This test can be used to monitor unaided recovery of self-regulation skills or to assess the efficacy of rehabilitation programs.
Social Support Questionnaire (SSQ; Sarason, Sarason, Shearin, & Pierce, 1987)	A 27-item assessment tool designed to measure individuals' perceptions of social support and their satisfaction with that support. Each item has two parts: listing individuals that fit the criteria and rating how satisfied they are with those people. It takes 5 minutes to administer.

(continued)

TABLE 5.1. *(continued)*

Tools	Description
Test of Everyday Attention (TEA; Robertson, Ward, Ridgeway, & Nimmo-Smith, 1994)*	A norm-referenced test of attention that uses functional activities in individuals ages 18–80 who have experienced an acquired neurological insult or who have attentional deficits (e.g., Asperger syndrome, ADHD, schizophrenia, myalgia, encephalomyelitis, HIV). The eight subtests involve everyday activities to identify the most important aspects of attention. It takes 90 minutes to administer and provide feedback.
Brief Resilience Scale (BRS; Smith et al., 2008)	A six-item survey tool that assess individuals' self-assessment of resiliency. More specifically, it identifies individuals' ability to recover from stress. This survey takes a few minutes to administer.
Ways of Coping Questionnaire (Folkman & Lazarus, 1988)	A 66-item questionnaire used to identify processes adults (i.e., high school through adulthood) use to cope with stressful situations. This test takes 10 minutes to administer.
Wechsler Test of Adult Reading (WTAR; Wechsler, 2001)*	A 50-item test of oral reading vocabulary that predicts verbal IQ in individuals ages 16–89. This test takes 10 minutes to administer.

Note. Asterisk (*) denotes tests of impairment.

the existing strategies are effective. Finding out what they believe (i.e., their self-efficacy and metacognitive beliefs) about their cognitive, communication, social life, test-taking and study skills, and time management and organization capabilities is an essential part of the coaching process. Students need to understand how they are perceiving their abilities and disabilities as a first step in self-discovery, and coaches need to know what students' believe since this will influence *how* they coach self-regulation and *where* they will start.

Besides supplemental tests, Table 5.1 includes several surveys and questionnaires that are useful for describing students' self-perceptions in important areas that are known to be related to academic and social aspects of college life, including:

- The ability to regulate one's own behavior and to think about one's thinking (metacognition) (e.g., the BRIEF-A: Behavior Rating Inventory of Executive Function—Adult; Roth et al., 2013).

- Social and coursework self-efficacy (e.g., CSEI: College Self-Efficacy Inventory—Solberg, O'Brien, Villareal, Kennel, & Davis, 1993; MSLQ: Motivational Studying and Learning Questionnaire—Pintrich & DeGroot, 1990).

- Social participation (e.g., MPAI-IV: Mayo–Portland Adaptability Inventory; Malec, 2005).

- General study strategies (e.g., LASSI: Learning and Study Strategies Inventory; Weinstein & Palmer, 2002).

- Resiliency (e.g., the BRS: Brief Resilience Scale; Smith et al., 2008).
- Coping abilities (e.g., WOC: Ways of Coping Questionnaire; Folkman & Lazarus, 1988).

In addition to these surveys and questionnaires, we developed the following three multipurpose survey tools: the College Survey for Students with Other Disabilities (CSS-OD; Kennedy, 2016; Form 5.4), the College Survey for Students with Brain Injury (CSS-BI; Kennedy & Krause, 2009; Form 5.5), and the College Survey for Students with Concussion (and Other Injuries) (CSS-CO; Kennedy, DeSalvio, & Nguyen, 2015). Note that the CSS-CO includes questions pertaining to other injuries, such as musculoskeletal injuries, but for our purposes here, it has been revised (in Form 5.6) to include questions pertinent to students with concussion only, and is referred to as the CSS-C. These surveys are similar in format and structure; they include a section on demographics, the history of injury and/or disability, the effects of the injury or disability, educational history, the services students have received and their perceived usefulness, and general questions about life changes (e.g., "Have you changed where you live? If yes, what was the change?"). Additionally, students are asked to rate their level of agreement (strongly disagree; disagree; neither agree nor disagree; agree; strongly agree) with statements that reflect academic and social experiences they have had. All three surveys share some common statements (e.g., "I have to review material more than I used to") and statements that are specific to the injury/disability. For example, the CSS-C contains statements that describe experiences of students with concussion (e.g., "I have trouble doing work on a computer or mobile device"), whereas the CSS-OD contains statements that reflect attentional control (e.g., "I get distracted in class").

In a large study of 103 individuals with and without TBI who had attended college, Kennedy, Krause, and O'Brien (2014) found that adults with TBI who reported more cognitive, psychosocial, and physical effects of the injury also reported more academic challenges. The exception was that, although more physical problems were reported by those with TBI, these problems did not predict the academic challenges they experienced, whereas cognitive and psychosocial problems did. Individuals with TBI also reported more academic challenges than did those without TBI. For those with TBI, an analysis of the relationships among the academic challenges revealed four primary groups of intercorrelations or domains: studying and learning, time management and organization, social challenges, and nervousness/stress/anxiety. This four-domain model accounted for a very large percentage (72%) of the variability. But there was overlap among some of these challenges. For example, for individuals with TBI, "being overwhelmed while studying" was related to studying and learning and to "being nervous before tests." For individuals without TBI, "being nervous before tests" was related to studying and learning only. In fact, for those without TBI, statements that included words such as "overwhelmed" were not related to anything that resembled being nervous or anxious, unlike those with TBI. Thus, we concluded that while studying and learning and time management and organization issues for individuals without TBI were similar in many ways to individuals with TBI, the psychological and social aspects interact differently when a student has a TBI. The CSS-C (Kennedy et al., 2015) is currently being validated in a study comparing college students with concussion to college students with other injuries, such as musculoskeletal injuries. Preliminary findings indicate that most college students with concussion report academic challenges that could be explained by their postconcussion physical and cognitive problems (e.g., fatigue, headaches, dizziness, trouble paying attention in class, forgetting what was said in class). Plans for validating the CSS-OD are under way.

From an earlier study of two college students with TBI (Kennedy & Krause, 2011) and from the results of the Kennedy and colleagues (2014) study we gained a better understanding of just how time management and organization, learning and studying, psychosocial concerns, and nervousness/anxiety were related. But how can students' responses to surveys and questionnaires be used to find out what they actually do when these situations arise? Semistructured interviews can do just that in the following ways:

- Verify and validate that students interpreted survey items as intended.
- Probe why students responded as they did.
- Determine what students do when these situations arise (i.e., what strategies or ways of coping do they engage in?).

We offer several forms that can guide coaches in how to use student responses as a starting point for semistructured interviews. Form 5.7 lists the academic statements about college students' experiences taken from the respective CSS surveys (CSS-OD, CSS-BI, and CSS-C). Since students will have already completed the entire survey, coaches can use these forms to have students rate how important their experiences are to them, which in turn provides valuable information to coaches about students' immediate priorities and what they are likely to be motivated to address first. Coaches then follow this up with open-ended questions, such as:

"Tell me more about this."

"What do you do when this happens?"

"Are there things you've tried in order to change this?"

"Do you use any strategies?"

It should be noted that the questions used in semistructured interviews can be used in conjunction with any of the survey tools listed in Table 5.1 and are not exclusive to the CSS tools. That being said, Table 5.2 provides an example of a conversation between a coach and a student about the student's perceptions, the importance of his or her experience, and the strategies being used, if any. This student endorses having to review material more and rates it as being important. However, the student is not sure about having fewer friends and does not consider this to be very important right now; another student may respond differently to this statement. It should also be noted that students' perceptions of these challenges and how important they are to them will likely change over time, as they adjust to the demands of college and the expectations of independence.

Notice the summary and open-ended statements by the coach that acknowledge the student's response, while asking for more details, followed by questions about describing what he or she does when this happens, and more specifically

TABLE 5.2. Using Students' Academic Challenges from the College Survey to Ask Deeper Questions about Strategies in a Semistructured Interview

Statement	Agreement rating (1 to 5)	Importance rating (1 to 5)	Category (MO, LS, SA, ST)	Interview questions: "Can you tell me more?"; "What do you do when this happens?"; "Are there things you've tried in order to change this?"; "Do you use any strategies?"; etc.
"I have to review material more than I used to."	5	4	LS	COACH: You definitely agree with this, and it's pretty important. Can you tell me more? STUDENT: I just have to work more at it. It takes me longer too. COACH: What do you do to review? Do you use any strategies? Do anything special? STUDENT: I read the book and highlight. Oh yeah, but now I have to highlight a lot more! COACH: Oh, OK. What do you highlight? STUDENT: Just about everything now. COACH: All right. Is there anything else you do? Other strategies? STUDENT: Mmm . . . not really. I just review the highlights.
"I have fewer friends than before."	3	1	SA	COACH: So you're not really sure that you have fewer friends. Is that right? STUDENT: Yeah, I don't really know what to expect from friends . . . I still have some buddies from high school that I hang with. I'm more focused on whether I can get back to where I was with my thinking, my memory, you know? COACH: Yup, I get that. This helps to know what your priorities are right now.

Note. MO, managing and organizing; LS, learning and studying; SA, self-advocacy; ST, stress, nervousness, anxiety.

about strategy use. This line of questioning is important. First, it allows the coach to acknowledge, in a nonjudgmental manner, the student's perceptions about a variety of academic challenges. Second, it gives the coach a better understanding of how the student interpreted the statement and the reasons for agreeing or disagreeing. Finally, questions about strategy use gives the coach critically important information about whether or not this student has strategies, whether or not strategies are used, and whether or not they are perceived as being effective. In the example given in Table 5.2, the coach discovers that the student is using ineffective highlighting strategies and spending a lot of time doing so. And because this is a high-priority area, the coach has a starting point for discussing more effective strategy options with the student as a part of the coaching plan. However, having more friends is not high priority for this student right now; it may become more of a priority later, after the student has experienced some academic success and has stronger self-efficacy around academic endeavors.

The CSS (-OD, -BI, -C) includes questions about students' use of campus services and other support services. Disability services, campus veterans services, groups for students with disabilities, and vocational rehabilitation services are some of the ones listed. Students are asked to indicate the extent to which they used these services and to also rate their usefulness. For example, students with brain injury or concussion may still be receiving rehabilitation services from a speech–language pathologist or occupational therapist and find these services very useful; however, they will impact their schedule and signals to the coach that others outside of the college campus will need to be team members as they begin to plan. Other students are not even aware that these services are available. Kennedy and colleagues (2008) found that nearly one-half of students with brain injury had never used or heard of campus disability services. When coaches ask students summary and open questions, student's usefulness ratings tell coaches about their perceptions of what worked, what did not, and why. The following example is one that is rather typical:

COACH: Can we review these a bit?

STUDENT: Sure.

COACH: So you went to disability services once?

STUDENT: Yeah, I went in the fall to register and get my accommodations letter.

COACH: OK, so have you been back since?

STUDENT: No, I just needed that letter.

COACH: And you think that has been somewhat useful. What do you mean?

STUDENT: Well, I got extended time—time and a half—for tests and assignments. And I can use a note taker. The notes help, but sometimes the student who I get notes from doesn't show up for class, so then I have to ask someone else. I mean, I don't know that many people in this class, and I just don't like asking so I don't always get the notes.

This line of questioning has revealed much more information than what could be obtained from relying solely on a student's ratings. From the above line of questioning, the coach discovers "what" the student is doing and "why" he or she is doing this (or not). Thus, the coach gets a deeper understanding of the student's behavior, which will help the coach support the student in the early phases of coaching:

• The student is not taking full advantage of disability services because he or she perceives them as offering little more than accommodations. It will be important to educate the student about the kinds of ongoing support that disability services can offer and explore his or her willingness to use these services. For example, accommodations can be changed if they are not working, although this requires that the student and the disability services provider have an established relationship. Students who have an ongoing relationship with their disability services provider are more likely to be able to get assistance such as modified accommodations, a reduction in courseload that is considered full time, and timely intervention when accommodations are not being implemented by instructors or teaching assistants.

• The student is hesitant to ask for assistance from peer note takers. A further conversation about the reasons could reveal that it is specific to this particular class; perhaps there are circumstances in this class that the student perceives as a barrier to requesting and getting good notes. However, it is also possible that the student does not want to call attention to his or her disability by asking for note takers. If this is the case, the coach and student could explore other ways to get notes, for example, having the instructor identify two peer note takers so that there is always a backup plan. This issue also may be a broader one of self-advocacy. It is possible that the student's reasons for not approaching note takers are similar to his or her reasons for visiting disability services only once—that the student is struggling with viewing him- or herself as someone who needs ongoing support, given that the student's real desire is to simply fit in with his or her peers. As this is often the case, discussions with the student about a willingness to use available supports will result in positive, real-life feedback while in college. Thus, positive changes in self-efficacy can occur with supportive coaching and positive everyday feedback that show students that they can succeed (Schmidt, Lannin, Fleming, & Ownsworth, 2011).

* The student reports only a few study strategies, such as highlighting and reviewing, which are passive and require little encoding. A discussion that explores more effective study strategies that the student could choose is warranted.

The CSS surveys also include open-ended questions about any major changes that have occurred because of a disability. Questions about living arrangements, academic majors, and changes in employment are located at the end of each survey. Students' responses provide coaches with rich information that signals that they may or may not have already seen the need for adjustments to their goals and pursuits because of their disabilities or that they are unsure whether or not their goals are realistic.

COLLABORATIVE PLANNING: TRANSLATION, GOAL WRITING, STUDENT OUTCOMES, AND INDIVIDUALIZED PLANS

Once the coach and student have collected information from tests, questionnaires, and surveys, the next step is to create a plan. In this section, we discuss three aspects of planning: (1) the translation of the clinical and educational results from reports into practical everyday examples that students can understand; (2) identifying multiple outcomes and various kinds of goals; (3) and creating individualized plans for coaching support.

Personalized Education: Translating Student Strengths and Challenges

Coaches with expertise in working with college students with TBI, concussion, and ADHD are particularly equipped to interpret and explain the factors underlying students' abilities and disabilities. Form 5.8 can be useful in guiding conversations about abilities and disabilities. Coaches may need to add some observations from test results to get the conversation going and may need to provide an example for the student. For instance, a student who has trouble initiating may be able to identify that this prevents him or her from starting projects, but not realize that it also prevents him from restarting a project after taking a break. Thus, a problem with initiation contributes to his or her ability to not just start, but to continue with, projects. In many cases, coaches will need to provide additional examples and use them to educate the student about how his or her underlying abilities and disabilities are observed.

Multiple Outcomes and Multiple Goals

When college students with executive function problems are asked, "What do you want to accomplish?," coaches get a wide variety of responses.

> "I want to get a B in calculus."
>
> "I want to turn papers in on time."
>
> "I want to graduate."
>
> "I want to see if I am going to be able to succeed in college."
>
> "I want to speak up more and ask questions in class."
>
> "I want to get to the point where I don't need disability services."
>
> "I want to figure out my major."
>
> "I want to share my injury experiences with high school students."
>
> "I want to meet more people."
>
> "I want to get better grades."

At first glance, these statements seem to have little in common and reflect a variety of outcomes that students want to achieve. But it's helpful to frame these student outcomes as goals that (1) are immediate, or "proximal," and long-range, or "distal," goals, (2) can be written as SMART(ER) goals with goal attainment scaling, and (3) emphasize self-regulation and performance-based outcomes.

Proximal goals are those that pertain to students' immediate needs as they relate to specific courses, work, friends, studying for exams, writing papers, and understanding and remembering what they read, for example. A proximal goal could be "I want to speak up more and ask questions in class" or "I want to get a B in calculus." Distal goals have the tendency to be vaguer and more difficult to measure (e.g., "I want to graduate"); they often need to be broken down into more proximal goals as a part of a larger plan. Distal goals can also be more difficult to achieve because time, experiences, and events can provide barriers over which students and/or coaches have little control.

Smarter Goals Using Goal Attainment Scaling

Most educators and rehabilitation specialists have been taught to create SMART goals because they contain important elements that can be easily operationalized. Though there are several variations of the elements of SMART goals, it is generally agreed that they be Specific, Measurable, Achievable, Realistic and/or Relevant, and Timed or Timely (McLellan, 1997). There are several online resources that provide step-by-step instructions for creating SMART goals. For example, Wake

Forest University provides brief definitions and examples of each of the elements of SMART (*http://professional.opcd.wfu.edu/files/2012/09/Smart-Goal-Setting.pdf*) that coaches can use to instruct students in how to create SMART goals. Hersh, Worral, Howe, Sherratt, and Davidson (2012) and Charles, Gafni, and Whelan (1999) emphasized the collaborative nature and shared decision making of goal setting. Here, SMARTER stands for Shared, Monitored, Accessible, Relevant, Transparent, Evolving, and Relationship-centered. Discussions that result in shared decision making is key in their approach. This latter version works nicely with our dynamic coaching model of collaboration.

Collaboration at this stage of coaching reinforces the MI principles of acceptance, encouragement, student autonomy, and trusting relationships. Additionally, the inclusion of "evolving" communicates that goals may very well need to be adjusted, and that students and coaches do not always know how feasible or realistic a goal really is until the steps to reach that goal are attempted. *A trusting relationship between coach and student creates opportunities for goals to change, rather than for unmet goals to be perceived as failures.* Students learn that setting goals and achieving them (or not) is a part of the self-regulation process, a means of self-discovery and self-efficacy. After all, if the student is the one carrying out the plan to achieve the goal, the student had better be involved in creating it. Using collaborative language in the form of acknowledgments and affirmations influences the likelihood that the individual will be able to identify the problem, the first step in setting goals (Hunt, Le Dorze, Polatajko, Bottari, & Dawson, 2015). In fact, goal setting can be undermined by "abrupt topic shifts, lack of acknowledgment and failure to explore what the client said" (p. 488).

Collaborative goal setting may be a shift for some coaches with a medical rehabilitation background. When clients are recovering from a brain injury and are receiving medically based rehabilitation services, they may not be capable of collaborating with clinicians in setting goals. However, as soon as clients have that capability, it is critical for clinicians to start engaging them in this process. As they recover and gain the cognitive skills and awareness (even as limited as that awareness might be), they can become partners in setting goals. Research has shown that when patients and clients are involved in setting personalized and practical goals, they are more likely to reach those goals because they have been a part of the goal-creation process (Kennedy, O'Brien, & Krause, 2012; Kennedy et al., 2008). For example, a discussion by the coach and student of the goal "I want to speak up more and ask questions in class" could focus on selecting the class for which this goal is fitting and achievable, on how often the student wants to speak up in class, and on how long the student wants to persist with this goal. After the discussion, the student's goal for herself could be "When given the opportunity in class, I will make a comment or ask a question at least once a week in each of my English and history classes this semester."

Goal attainment scaling (GAS) is a method of goal writing that quantifies individuals' personal interpretation of what it means to make progress toward achieving the goal (Kiresuk & Sherman, 1968; Kiresuk, Smith, & Cardillo, 2013). Rating scales are used to describe the degree to which the goal is being met. Traditionally, a score of 0 is the starting point, or "baseline," and movement up and down the scale represents improvement toward meeting and even exceeding the goal (e.g., +1, +2), or regressing and performing worse than where the individual started (e.g., –1, –2). Rating scales can also use descriptors rather than numbers, such as "the same," "better," or "worse."

Both educators and rehabilitation professionals have worked with GAS, so coaches from these backgrounds should be fairly familiar with it. For example, school counselors have used GAS to document the outcomes after student and counselor consultations (Brady, Busse, & Lopez, 2014). However, to make sure that goals are reliable and valid, GAS should be used in conjunction with the SMART goal structure. An international group of clinical researchers has described some concerns with the use of GAS, mainly that its reliability and validity are dependent on the individuals who created it (Krasny-Pacini, Evans, Sohlberg, & Chevignard, 2016). A sample of a SMARTER goal using GAS is provided in Chapter 6.

Deciding which rating scale to use depends on the student. Many students do not object to using negative numbers to indicate that they fall below the starting point; however, others do, so we more often use a +2 as the starting point. Giving students both options and having them select their rating scale of choice will increase the likelihood that they will follow through with tracking their performance since they will have identified the kind of feedback (positive or negative) that will motivate them. Form 5.9 provides coaches and students with templates for creating SMARTER goals using GAS.

Performance Goals and Self-Regulation Goals

How coaches create SMARTER goals using GAS with students is only part of the goal-generation process. Most professionals are trained to write what we call "performance-based "goals. For example, a SMARTER goal might read as "I will keep up with all of the assigned readings in my three courses this semester" or "I will turn in completed assignments on time in my three courses this semester." Both of these goals are specific, can be measured, are realistic, are defined by a finite time frame, and may be achievable. Yet, to reach these goals, students must go through a series of self-regulation steps, implementing each step along the way. For students with executive function problems, these steps are a challenge.

Performance-based goals are appealing when they rely on the SMARTER components; however, they are typically the end result of *several intermediate self-regulation steps are required in order to be achieved.* Performance-based goals target only the level of the skill and implicit changes in self-regulation; they do not explicitly activate the self-regulation process that facilitates an updated understanding and deepening self-efficacy of the skill. If coaches are going to instruct students in self-regulation, then self-regulation goals need to be explicit. Each component of self-regulation (goals, strategies, implementing, and adjusting) is associated with a number of steps, any one of which can become goals themselves, if that is the part of the self-regulation process in which the student is struggling. Figure 4.2 in Chapter 4 identifies the various steps in self-regulation. By targeting the specific part of the process that is challenging for the student, coaches can explicitly instruct students in how to self-regulate for a wide variety of skills.

"The student will recall four out of five details from orally presented stories after a 5-minute delay across three sessions" is a performance-based goal. However, this goal tells us nothing about *how* the student accomplished this. In order to reach performance goals, students must select and then implement strategies and plans, and then decide if the goal was met. If a student does not have a useful strategy or has one but does not use it, then it is unlikely that the performance goal will be achieved. Thus, performance-based goals tell us nothing about why or how the goal was achieved. What strategies were used? How much time, practice, and effort did it take to learn the strategy? Did the student attempt to adjust the strategy? Is a 5-minute delay sufficient to ensure later recall, which is the real goal of learning? What is the likelihood that the strategy used here will be generalized or transfer to other kinds of learning?

Take a student with time-management problems, whose goals are to keep up with weekly readings and turn in assignments on time. The first example in Table 5.3 shows the student's performance goals and the problems faced by the student who does not really know how much time it takes him or her to read and complete

TABLE 5.3. Examples of How Self-Regulation and Performance Goals Are Generated and Are Related to Each Other

Student goal	Coaching follow-up	Example self-regulation goals	Example performance goals
"I want to keep up in class." → Student responds: "It should only take 2 hours to do the assigned readings, but I'm not really sure . . . so how can I plan? I'm worried about getting assignments done on time too." "Sure."	"Tell me more about that. Describe for me what's happening." → "OK, would you be willing to track how much time it's taking you compared to how long you think it will take?" → Coach instructs student in "plan–do–review" and provides form.	1. Student will accurately assess how long it takes to read. 2. Student will accurately assess how long it takes to complete an assignment.	1. Student will keep up with the readings this semester. 2. Student will turn in assignments on time this semester.

assignments. Because the time involved for these tasks is not known, two simi-lar self-regulation goals are warranted. Both target predicting how much time it will take him or her to read and to complete assignments. These steps are critical because without knowing how much time these tasks take, neither the coach nor the student can create strategies or plans to reach his performance-based goals. After some discussion, the student agrees to address these self-regulation goals first, by predicting and tracking the time it takes to read and complete assignments. A comparison of these two shows that it took the student longer to complete these kinds of activities than he had thought. With these results in hand, the coach and student can then begin to make adjustments in his schedule so that the student can reach the goals of keeping up with readings and turning in assignments on time.

Thus, there are a number of advantages to establishing self-regulation, as opposed to performance, goals:

1. Self-regulation goals target the process that students go through to problem-solve and learn what will work (or not work) in order to achieve their final performance goal.

2. Self-regulation goals are often attainable even when performance goals are not. For example, students who learn how long it takes them to read assign-ments have gained a deeper understanding of the impact of their disability. ven if they don't always keep up with the reading (a performance goal), the information gained from this process will help them plan on a weekly, monthly, and semester basis.

3. Gaining information about how the underlying self-regulation process works allows students to generalize self-regulation steps to future classes and semesters.

4. Self-regulation goals emphasize students' choice; students play an active role in their own problem solving by suggesting strategies, evaluating their effectiveness, and making adjustments.

5. Self-regulation goals create opportunities for students to monitor their own progress. The self-regulation process places the responsibility for reaching their goals squarely with the students themselves. Coaches support and instruct up to a point, but students must be active partners.

Documenting Other Outcomes When Coaching Self-Regulation

College students with executive function problems will mature and change, as do college students without disabilities. Speech–language pathologists, neuropsy-chologists, educators, occupational therapists, and vocational rehabilitation coun-selors may need to document progress in ways that are required by third-party payers. While student-centered goals are a necessity for students who are enrolled in college, there are other kinds of outcomes that validate the usefulness of coaching self-regulation (e.g., Lichtinger & Kaplan, 2015). Here we highlight three kinds of outcomes: grades and test scores, self-regulation outcomes from surveys and questionnaires, and changes in distal, or long-term, goals.

Improved grades on class assignments, quizzes, and exams are obviously expected by students and coaches. Immediate positive changes on graded assignments are not only validating for students who implemented strategies and plans in which they were coached, but these changes also have a positive impact on students' long-range goals of succeeding in college and eventually graduating. Implementing strategies and plans and then experiencing positive outcomes are both rewarding and motivating; students who get initial positive feedback in reaching their goals are more likely to persevere as they gain self-efficacy. Kennedy and Krause (2011) reported that two students with TBI made immediate improvement in graded assignments while being coached. However, changes in grades may also reflect the end result of going through the self-regulation process. Even though students want better grades, coaches want them to know how to best go about it. Again, one student with TBI stated, "Oh, I get it, you want me to become my own coach!"

Documenting changes in self-regulation is made easier by using survey responses and questionnaires that are psychometrically solid. Several kinds of positive changes have been reported during or after dynamic coaching. Kennedy and Krause (2011) reported that changes in ratings that signify improved perception or acknowledgment can be used to document deeper self-awareness. Some students reported that they used more strategies, and others admitted using a larger variety of strategies. O'Brien, Schellinger, and Kennedy (2017) coded strategies that were elicited during semistructured interviews in response to the students ratings of their academic challenges on Form 5.7 for college students with brain injury. They found that after coaching, college students with TBI reported using a wider repertoire of studying, learning, and time-management strategies categorized by Zimmerman and Martinez-Pons (1986). In other words, students had broadened their repertoire of tools. The effectiveness of coaching was corroborated by improved grades and reports of less stress, nervousness, and frustration. Other practical changes include accessing and rating the usefulness of campus services, such as student disability services, campus counseling services, and veterans campus centers, can be documented using tools such as the College Students with Disabilities Campus Climate survey (CSDCC; Lombardi, Gerdes, & Murray (2011) or the CSS-OD (Form 5.4), CSS-BI (Form 5.5), or CSS-C (Form 5.6).

Other outcomes are more distal, or long term. Semistructured interview questions that are open ended with respect to choosing majors and plans for graduation, careers, living arrangements, and so forth, can also be attributed in part to coaching, with the caution that all college students change over time. If students explicitly attribute some of these decisions to the coaching support that they received, then it is fair to say that dynamic coaching played an important role. As one student stated, "My coach helped me see and experience what I *could* do, not just what I couldn't do. And that helped me decide on my major." Finally, tools like the Brief Resilience Scale (Smith et al., 2008), the Social Support Questionnaire (Sarason, Sarason, Shearin, & Pierce, 1987), and the College Self-Efficacy Inventory (Solberg et al., 1993) can document changes in students' ability to bounce back, to expand their social network, and to strengthen their self-efficacy.

Individualized Plans

Now that information has been gathered and goals have been discussed, it is time for the coach and student to integrate these processes into a coherent plan. The plan needs to be clear enough for the student and coach to follow, so that the student has in mind how his or her immediate academic needs are being addressed as the semester progresses, while keeping in mind the more distal or long-term outcomes. Concrete, written plans are helpful also in documenting progress. From week to week, it is easy to slip into focusing on urgent or current needs only, but explicitly viewing how those needs fit into a larger plan will help students understand how proximal goals will fit into distal goals.

On the other hand, students will be reporting successes and challenges, and training in self-regulation focuses on how the student adjusts over time. This means that just as strategies may change to address a student's needs or priorities, goals may also need to be adjusted, and it is reasonable to expect and even *plan* for changes to the plan. Students need to know that this kind of adjustment is expected and will be managed in conjunction with the coach. For example, after one semester of coaching, one student realized that his goal of a 4.0 average was unrealistic and was preventing him from socializing with his roommates. He modified his goal to a 3.5 and set an additional goal to participate in one social activity each week. The plan changed in conjunction with this updating of goals, so that social communication and advocacy were included as well as academic needs.

The plan contains enough detail for the student and coach to know what should be addressed across the course of the semester, but it is not unnecessarily detailed with specifics about strategies or tools that may be used. Essentially, the plan is developed by collecting goals into categories and organizing them into a coherent sequence based on when they should be addressed. Remember that goals are centered around three types of outcomes:

1. *Proximal* academic goals, like grades on assignments and test scores.
2. *Self-regulation* outcomes from rating scales and forms, surveys, and questionnaires.
3. *Distal,* or long-term, goals, like graduating on time.

Plans are also developed around the way goals are organized. This format is logical for students because academic performance is paired with self-regulation goals, and these, in turn, advance students' long-term goals.

Students and coaches might find it helpful to begin planning by taking a "triage" approach. Items may have been identified as being particularly important when goals were initially set, but may not be relevant to what students need now. Coaches can question students about immediate needs such as:

"Are you making it to classes on time? Are you comfortable with your schedule?"

"Are you experiencing academic failures?"

"Do you have a plan to implement accommodations provided by disability services?"

"Do you know what you need to do this week? Next week?"

"Are there tests or assignments due this week?"

In some cases, the semester may have started, and students may already be struggling in courses before coaching is initiated. For students with acquired injuries or newly diagnosed students who had been successful in structured secondary educational settings, the newness of the academic failures can be particularly distressing. Students may feel at a loss to know how to manage their studying and learning if they received a failing grade on a test or assignment. Similarly, if students are struggling to manage their daily schedules or are unsure when and where they need to be for classes or about how to manage transportation (parking, bus schedules, carpooling, etc.), then these needs should be addressed first.

However, it is unlikely that these kinds of difficulties will be "new" information discovered when developing the plan. Those needs—such as difficulty with tests or managing a daily schedule—should have been identified during information gathering, and goals should have been put in place. Here, those goals are being triaged by immediacy. If students are experiencing academic failure, the plan should be changed immediately to address those needs first. In a similar vein, if students are struggling to arrive to class on time or to even know what and when assignments are due, then academic issues cannot be addressed until time-management and organization needs are managed.

Therefore, the plan should be developed based on:

- The student's immediate needs (issues to be resolved in the next week).
- Proximal goals (achievable within the semester or academic year) paired with self-regulation goals.
- Distal (long-term) goals.

Students may benefit from seeing these goals described in a time-ordered sequence. Figure 5.2 shows how one student's goals were structured with respect to the student's needs and how the plan progressed. Note that these goals are all performance based and are written in language that the student might have used, or at the least, that the student can easily understand and follow. Students rarely use the language of self-regulation in describing their needs (e.g., "I need to stop procrastinating and get my work done on time," rather than, "I need to monitor my Internet and Netflix usage, particularly before assignments are due"). Instead, the goals describing monitoring and strategy adjustment (as part of self-regulation)

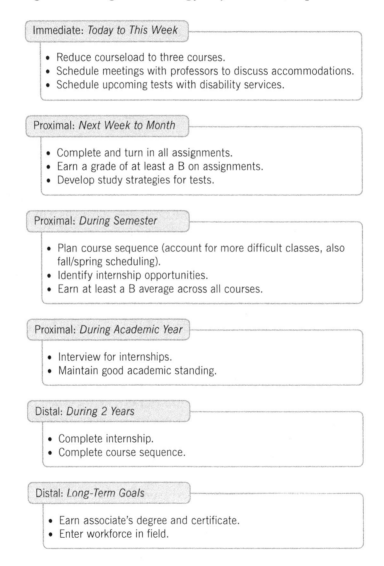

Immediate: *Today to This Week*

- Reduce courseload to three courses.
- Schedule meetings with professors to discuss accommodations.
- Schedule upcoming tests with disability services.

Proximal: *Next Week to Month*

- Complete and turn in all assignments.
- Earn a grade of at least a B on assignments.
- Develop study strategies for tests.

Proximal: *During Semester*

- Plan course sequence (account for more difficult classes, also fall/spring scheduling).
- Identify internship opportunities.
- Earn at least a B average across all courses.

Proximal: *During Academic Year*

- Interview for internships.
- Maintain good academic standing.

Distal: *During 2 Years*

- Complete internship.
- Complete course sequence.

Distal: *Long-Term Goals*

- Earn associate's degree and certificate.
- Enter workforce in field.

FIGURE 5.2. Examples of mapping proximal and distal goals onto a plan by immediacy of need.

typically develop during MI. Form 5.10 is a chart that helps coaches keep track of these various kinds of goals, and Form 5.11 is a chart that helps students write down and prioritize goals based on immediacy of need.

Because students should have already met with disability services and have arranged accommodations, coaches should begin by reviewing these accommodations and having students describe how they will be implemented. You may note that this student's most immediate needs were situated around managing accommodations provided by disability services and in reducing the courseload before the semester deadline to drop a class. The student was unsure how to approach his professors to present his letter of accommodations from disability services. He had considered approaching his professors after classes, but had found that other students were also waiting and he felt uncomfortable discussing his learning needs with a group of his peers listening in. After receiving the syllabi on the first day of classes, this student also realized that taking four courses was unrealistic, particularly in light of his academic goal to maintain a B average. The student was also taking a difficult biology course, an unfamiliar subject that semester, and needed to dedicate extra time toward succeeding in that class. The plan reflects the timeline of these needs, allowing the student to adjust his courseload to match his goals and put accommodations in place, then moving on to goals that can be addressed over several weeks.

Samples of self-regulation plans and goals that can be paired with this student's proximal goals are shown in Figure 5.3. This student was performing poorly in school, but after reviewing the student's work, it became clear that the

---

Self-Regulation Proximal Goals: *Next Week to Month*

- **Complete and turn in all assignments.**
  - Develop planner to manage assignments.
    - Identify necessary features of planner, pilot tool, and adjust as necessary.
    - Describe process to check accuracy of planner (with syllabus and classnotes).
  - Develop process to track accuracy of assignment completion.
    - Track accuracy of assignment completion using an online gradebook, checking folders for assignments, and planner for checkboxes.
- **Earn a grade of at least a B on all assignments.**
  - Complete all assignments on time.
  - Accurately monitor time to completion to allow for editing and proofreading as needed.
- **Develop study strategies for tests.**
  - Use reading journal to recall read material.
    - Assess if notes are effective in triggering recall.
  - Plan ahead to allow for studying for tests over time.
    - Check accuracy of time estimation for studying.
  - Use multiple strategy approach for memorization.
    - Determine strategies most effective for recall.

FIGURE 5.3. Sample self-regulation goals to pair with proximal goals.

student was forgetting to turn in assignments. Therefore, self-regulation goals first focused on developing a system to monitor assignment completion, then focused on addressing learning and studying needs. This component of the plan meshes with and specifies how proximal goals will be met.

Students and coaches should also discuss whether specific classes versus general learning will be targeted. Needs for classes vary widely. For example, a student may have required reading for all his or her courses, but that reading will be different if it is for a course in chemistry, statistics, world history, or the English novel. Some classes play to students' strengths or weaknesses as well. Classes in a student's major may be more rigorous, but the student's base of knowledge in that area may make these classes less challenging than those in related fields. Other classes may challenge executive function, in particular, like courses that have several long-term projects that need to be organized and planned to be completed over a period of time. Students may choose to focus their efforts on these selected courses, such as tailoring reading strategies for novels or memorization for physics.

The final step in generating a plan now that the sequence of goals has been laid out is to decide the amount and type of support that will be appropriate for students to both meet their goals and to become independent managers of their learning. Most students choose to meet with coaches weekly, at least during the first semester, so that the meeting becomes part of their academic routine. Students also find that such regularly scheduled meetings "keep them persisting," meaning that if they know they need to meet with their coach to talk about their plans and strategies, then they are more likely to have kept up with their work. However, the student and coach can settle on the schedule of meetings that best suits the student's needs.

Now that you know how to gather the necessary information from students about their strengths and weaknesses and how to coach them to create both self-regulation and performance-based goals, let's turn to three specific areas that college students with executive function problems need support in: time management and organization, studying and learning, and self-advocacy. Chapter 6 provides you with coaching practices that use the GSAA approach for the first two domains, and Chapter 7 provides you with an understanding of and coaching practices for the last domain, self-advocacy.

Getting Started Checklist for Coaches

Here is a list of documents that you will need to get to know a student, assess a student's abilities and disabilities, and begin to create a coaching plan. Most of these documents should be provided by the student him- or herself.

☐ Form 4.1, What to Expect with Dynamic Coaching (to be sent to the student).

☐ An unofficial copy of the student's college and/or high school transcripts.

☐ A list of courses in which the student is currently enrolled

☐ A letter from the student's disability service specialist that authorizes and lists the reasonable accommodations that the student is entitled to receive, if available.

☐ Reports by psychologists and other professionals who tested the student's cognitive, communication, and vocational skills.

☐ A list of supplemental tests that will need to be administered.

☐ Form 5.3, Demographic, Academic, Medical, and Social History Form (to be completed by the student)

☐ Questionnaires and surveys, such as Form 5.4, College Survey for Students with Other Disabilities; Form 5.5, College Survey for Students with Brain Injury; and Form 5.6, College Survey for Students with Concussion (to be completed by the student).

☐ Contact information for any other professionals who are providing care or support to the student.

☐ Name of the planner or scheduling system that the student uses.

Getting Started Checklist for Students

Instructions: The first coaching session involves gathering information to review and plan what you and your coach will be working on over the semester and/or year. Please bring these documents with you to the first coaching session:

☐ A copy of Form 4.1, What to Expect with Dynamic Coaching, and any questions you may have.

☐ An unofficial copy of your college and/or high school transcripts.

☐ Reports by neuropsychologists and/or other professionals who have tested your cognitive, communication, and vocational skills.

☐ A letter from your disability service specialist, if available, that authorizes and lists the reasonable accommodations that you are entitled to receive.

☐ Completed Form 5.____, College Survey for Students with _____.

☐ Other additional questionnaires that the coach sent to you to complete

☐ Completed Form 5.3, Demographic, Academic, Medical, and Social History Form.

☐ Contact information for any other professionals from whom you are receiving support or assistance.

☐ A list of current courses.

☐ The planner or scheduling system you use.

Demographic, Academic, Medical, and Social History Form

DEMOGRAPHIC INFORMATION

Name: _____ Date: _____

Address: _____

Phone numbers: Home: _____ Mobile: _____

Email address: _____

Date of birth: _____

Do you speak and understand more than one language? (Circle)   Yes   No

- Which language is your primary one? _____

Do you currently live independently from your family? (Circle)   Yes   No

ACADEMIC AND MEDICAL HISTORY

When you were in elementary, middle, or high school, did you have any difficulty learning how to read or write? (Circle)   Yes   No

If yes, explain: _____

_____

_____

_____

Did you ever receive assistance in school in the form of speech therapy, remedial help, or special education? (Circle)   Yes   No

If yes, explain: _____

_____

_____

_____

If you are in college now, what kind of grades have you received? _____

_____

- About how many college credits have you completed? _____
- What is your college major, if you have one? _____
- What do you hope to do after you graduate? _____

(continued)

Have you ever been diagnosed with, or been told that you have, the following conditions? If yes, include the dates when this condition first occurred.

Diagnosis	No	Yes	Explanation, dates
Stroke			
Cancer or tumor			
Multiple sclerosis			
Traumatic brain injury, including concussion			
Posttraumatic stress disorder (PTSD)			
Seizures			
Attention-deficit disorder or attention-deficit/hyperactivity disorder			
Learning disability: if so, what kind?			
Intellectual disability			
Autism spectrum disorder			
Other kind of neurological problems			
Other physical problems (e.g., mobility, vision, hearing)			

Have you ever been diagnosed with clinical depression, anxiety, stress disorder, bipolar disorder, or other mental health diagnoses? (Circle)   Yes   No

If yes, explain: _____

_____

List all of the medications you are currently taking.

_____ for _____

_____ for _____

_____ for _____

_____ for _____

(continued)

SOCIAL HISTORY

What do you do for fun? _____

_____

- Do you do these activities with other people? (Circle)   Yes   No

    Explain: _____

    _____

How many times a week do you get together with friends? _____

How many times a week do you get together with family? _____

Do you stay in touch with friends from high school? (Circle)   Yes   No

- Explain how important or unimportant this is to you: _____

    _____

Are you involved in any organizations on or off campus, like chorus, athletics, chess, or nonprofit groups, etc.? (Circle)   Yes   No

If yes, what kind? _____

_____

Do you use social media to stay in touch with friends or family? (Circle)   Yes   No

If yes, how many times a day are you on social media? _____

- Has spending time on social media sites ever interfered with getting other things done? (Circle)   Yes   No

    If yes, explain: _____

    _____

Do you drink alcohol? (Circle)   Yes   No

If yes, how much and how often? _____

- Have you received rehabilitation or help for alcohol abuse? (Circle)   Yes   No

    If yes, explain: _____

    _____

Do you use recreational or other drugs? (Circle)   Yes   No

If yes, how much and how often? _____

- Have you received rehabilitation or help for drug abuse? (Circle)   Yes   No

    If yes, explain: _____

    _____

(continued)

ADDITIONAL QUESTIONS FOR STUDENTS WHO HAVE HAD A TBI (INCLUDING CONCUSSION), STROKE, MULTIPLE SCLEROSIS, PTSD, OR OTHER ACQUIRED INJURIES

Were you ever unconscious? (Circle)   Yes   No

If yes, for how long? _____

_____

Were you hospitalized? (Circle)   Yes   No

If yes, for how long? _____

_____

Did you receive rehabilitation, as an inpatient or an outpatient? (Circle)   Yes   No

If yes, for how long? _____

_____

Had you attended college before this happened? (Circle)   Yes   No

If so, how much college had you completed? _____

- Have you returned to college? (Circle)   Yes   No
- Did you take time off from college before returning? (Circle)   Yes   No

   If yes, how much time off? _____

   _____

Were you working at the time this happened? (Circle)   Yes   No

If yes, what kind of work? _____

- Did you take time off from work? (Circle)   Yes   No

   If yes, how much time off from work? _____

   _____

- Have you returned to work? (Circle)   Yes   No
- If yes, are you doing the same job and getting paid the same amount? (Circle)   Yes   No

   If yes, explain: _____

   _____

College Survey for Students with Other Disabilities (CSS-OD)

Name: _____ Date: _____

Coach: _____

Instructions: Please complete this form as best you can. Your coach will review it with you as well.

I. Demographics

Date of birth: _____

Sex: (Circle)   Female   Male

Are you currently enrolled in college? (Circle)   Yes   No

If yes, how many years of college have you completed? (Circle)   1   2   3   4   5   6   7+

When did you start college? Provide the date: _____

II. Type of Disability

What type(s) of disability do you have, and how old were you when it was discovered? Circle your answer. If yes, at what age?					
Attention-deficit disorder or attention-deficit/hyperactivity disorder	Yes	No	0–11	12–17	18+
Learning disability: reading and/or writing	Yes	No	0–11	12–17	18+
Learning disability: math and/or spatial relations	Yes	No	0–11	12–17	18+
Intellectual disability	Yes	No	0–11	12–17	18+
Autism spectrum disorder	Yes	No	0–11	12–17	18+
Other (please specify):	Yes	No	0–11	12–17	18+

(continued)

III. Other Factors

Check all that apply, and indicate whether you have ever received therapy for each effect.		
	Experienced the effect	Had therapy for the effect
Problems making decisions		
Difficulty with relationships		
Physical impairment: arm/hands (writing, etc.)		
Mood changes		
Anger		
Physical impairment: legs (walking, etc.)		
Substance/alcohol abuse		
Memory problems		
Dizziness		
Headaches		
Attention problems		
Fatigue		
Organization problems		
Depression		
Difficulty maintaining friendships		
Physical impairment: vision		
Difficulty with academics, like studying, homework, tests		
Physical impairment: hearing		
Other (specify):		

IV. Support or Therapies for Disability

Which of the following have you received? Circle your answer.			
Psychological counseling	None	Past (completed)	Ongoing/current
Physical therapy	None	Past (completed)	Ongoing/current
Speech or language therapy	None	Past (completed)	Ongoing/current
Occupational therapy	None	Past (completed)	Ongoing/current
Peer support group	None	Past (completed)	Ongoing/current

(continued)

126

Which of the following have you received? Circle your answer.			
Vocational counseling	None	Past (completed)	Ongoing/current
Accommodations in school	None	Past (completed)	Ongoing/current
What kind of accommodations have you had?			
Special education when in elementary, middle, and/or high school	None	Past (completed)	Ongoing/current
What kind of special education did you receive?			

V. Your Student Experiences

To what extent do you agree with each of the following statements about your experience as a student? If you have *attended college, consider your experiences since you've been in college.*	Strongly disagree	Disagree	Neither agree nor disagree	Agree	Strongly agree
I procrastinate on things I need to do.					
I get overwhelmed when studying.					
I get overwhelmed in class.					
I get nervous before tests.					
I have trouble managing my time.					
I am late to class.					
I have trouble meeting deadlines.					
I have trouble prioritizing assignments.					
Others do not understand my problems.					
I forget what has been said in class.					
I have fewer friends than I thought I would have.					
I don't always understand instructions for assignments.					
I get distracted while studying.					
I have to review material more than I thought I would.					
I get distracted in class.					
I don't know how to start large projects.					
The assignments I turn in are messy or disorganized.					
I get impatient when working in groups.					

(continued)

To what extent do you agree with each of the following statements about your experience as a student? If you have *attended college, consider your experiences since you've been in college.*					
	Strongly disagree	Disagree	Neither agree nor disagree	Agree	Strongly agree
I have trouble understanding what I read in textbooks.					
I get frustrated easily.					
I forget what friends or family tell me.					
I tend to say what I think regardless of the situation.					
I have trouble following through on things I say I will do.					
I don't socialize with friends as much as I would like.					
Are you interested in meeting other students with similar disabilities? (Circle) Yes No					
Are you interested in getting help from a specialist in working with college students with these disabilities? (Circle) Yes No					

VI. Your Use of Services

If you have attended college, indicate the extent to which you have used these services.						
	Never heard of it	Heard of it, but never used	Once	Sometimes	Pretty often	All the time
Campus disability services						
Campus veterans' services						
Campus counseling services						
Campus medical services						
Campus group for students with disabilities						
Campus tutoring or academic center						
State vocational rehabilitation services						
Community-based services						
Specify any other services you have received:						

(continued)

VII. Rating Services

For *any service that you have used at least once,* indicate how useful you found the service.	Completely useless	Somewhat useless	Somewhat useful	Extremely useful	N/A
Campus disability services					
Campus veterans' services					
Campus counseling services					
Campus medical services					
Campus group for students with disabilities					
Campus tutoring or academic center					
State vocational rehabilitation services					
Community-based services					
Specify any other services you have received:					

VIII. Life Changes

Identify any changes you have made in your life plans, goals, work situation, etc., because of your disability. If you have no college experience yet, answer these questions as best you can.	
Have you changed what college or university you attend? If yes, what did you change it from and to?	Circle: Yes/No Explain:
Have you changed your academic major? If yes, what was the change?	Circle: Yes/No Explain:
Have you changed your academic status (e.g., full time vs. part time)? If yes, what was the change?	Circle: Yes/No Explain:
Have you changed your career goal(s)? If yes, what was the change?	Circle: Yes/No Explain:
Have you changed where you live? If yes, what was the change?	Circle: Yes/No Explain:
Have you changed your current employment? If yes, what was the change?	Circle: Yes/No Explain:
Other comments:	

College Survey for Students with Brain Injury (CSS-BI)

Name: _____ Date: _____

Coach: _____

Instructions: Please complete this form as best you can. Your coach will review it with you as well.

I. Demographics

Fill in the following: (MM/DD/YYYY)

Date of birth ____/____/_____

Date of brain injury (estimate if you are not certain) ____/____/_____

Sex: (Circle)   Female   Male

Are you currently enrolled in college? (Circle)   Yes   No

How many years of college have you completed? (Circle)   1   2   3   4   5   6   7+

What years were you or have been enrolled in college? (e.g., 2000–2004; 2014 to current)

II. Type of Brain Injury

What type(s) of brain injury do you have, and how old were you when each occurred? Circle your answer.		
	Did you have this type of injury?	If yes, at what age?
Traumatic brain injury (TBI)	Yes No	0–11 12–17 18+
Stroke	Yes No	0–11 12–17 18+
Brain tumor	Yes No	0–11 12–17 18+
Multiple sclerosis (MS)	Yes No	0–11 12–17 18+
Parkinson's disease (PD)	Yes No	0–11 12–17 18+
Encephalitis	Yes No	0–11 12–17 18+
Other (please specify)	Yes No	0–11 12–17 18+

(continued)

Reprinted with permission from Mary R. T. Kennedy and Miriam O. Krause (2009).

III. History of Injury

Answer the following questions. Circle your answer.		
	Yes/no/don't know	If yes, approximately how long?
Were you in the hospital after your injury?	Yes/no/don't know	Semester(s): 1 2 3 4 Day(s): 1 2 3 4 5 6 Week(s): 1 2 3 Month(s): 1 2 3 4 5 6 7 8 9 10 11 Year(s) 1 Ongoing, N/A, Other
Were you unconscious or in a coma after your injury?	Yes/no/don't know	Semester(s): 1 2 3 4 Day(s): 1 2 3 4 5 6 Week(s): 1 2 3 Month(s): 1 2 3 4 5 6 7 8 9 10 11 Year(s) 1 Ongoing, N/A, Other
Did you, or are you now, receiving any therapy or rehabilitation after your injury?	Yes/no/don't know	Semester(s): 1 2 3 4 Day(s): 1 2 3 4 5 6 Week(s): 1 2 3 Month(s): 1 2 3 4 5 6 7 8 9 10 11 Year(s) 1 Ongoing, N/A, Other
Did you take a break from work or school after your injury?	Yes/no/don't know	Semester(s): 1 2 3 4 Day(s): 1 2 3 4 5 6 Week(s): 1 2 3 Month(s): 1 2 3 4 5 6 7 8 9 10 11 Year(s) 1 Ongoing, N/A, Other
Is brain injury your primary disability (choose "N/A" for length of time)	Yes/no/don't know	Semester(s): 1 2 3 4 Day(s): 1 2 3 4 5 6 Week(s): 1 2 3 Month(s): 1 2 3 4 5 6 7 8 9 10 11 Year(s) 1 Ongoing, N/A, Other
If you stated Other for a length of time, explain here:		

(continued)

IV. Effects of Brain Injury

What have been some effects of your brain injury? Check all that apply, and indicate whether you have ever received therapy for each effect.

	Experienced the effect	Had therapy for the effect
Difficulty with academics, like studying, homework, tests		
Problems making decisions		
Difficulty with relationships		
Physical impairment: arm/hands (writing, etc.)		
Mood changes		
Anger		
Physical impairment: legs (e.g., walking)		
Substance/alcohol abuse		
Memory problems		
Dizziness		
Headaches		
Attention problems		
Fatigue		
Organization problems		
Depression		
Difficulty maintaining friendships		
Other (specify):		

V. Support or Therapies for Brain Injury

Which of the following therapies have you received *because* of your brain injury? Circle your answer.

Psychological counseling	None Past (completed) Ongoing/current
Physical therapy	None Past (completed) Ongoing/current
Speech or language therapy	None Past (completed) Ongoing/current
Occupational therapy	None Past (completed) Ongoing/current
Support group	None Past (completed) Ongoing/current
Vocational counseling	None Past (completed) Ongoing/current
If other, specify:	

(continued)

VI. Your Student Experiences

To what extent do you agree with each of the following statements about your experience as a college student *since your brain injury*?	Strongly disagree	Disagree	Neither agree nor disagree	Agree	Strongly agree
I procrastinate on things I need to do.					
I get overwhelmed when studying.					
I get overwhelmed in class.					
I get nervous before tests.					
I have trouble managing my time.					
I am late to class.					
I have trouble prioritizing assignments and meeting deadlines.					
Others do not understand my problems.					
I forget what has been said in class.					
I have fewer friends than before.					
I don't always understand instructions for assignments.					
I have trouble paying attention in class or while studying.					
I have to review material more than I used to.					
Are you interested in meeting other students with brain injury? (Circle) Yes or No					
Are you interested in getting help from an educational specialist in brain injury? (Circle) Yes or No					

VII. Your Use of Services

Since you have been in college (or when you were in college), did you use the following services because of your brain injury?	Never heard of it	Heard of it, but never used	Once	Sometimes	Pretty often	All the time
Campus disability services						
Campus veterans' services						
Campus counseling services						
Campus medical services						
Campus group for students with disabilities						
State brain injury association						

(continued)

	Never heard of it	Heard of it, but never used	Once	Sometimes	Pretty often	All the time
State vocational rehabilitation services						
Other hospital or rehabilitation services						
If other, specify; or write any other comments here.						

VIII. Rating Services

For *any service that you have used at least once*, indicate how useful you found the service.					
	Completely useless	Somewhat useless	Somewhat useful	Extremely useful	N/A
Campus disability services					
Campus veterans' services					
Campus counseling services					
Campus medical services					
Campus group for students with disabilities					
State brain injury association					
State vocational rehabilitation services					
Other hospital or rehabilitation services					
If other, specify; or write any other comments here.					

(continued)

IX. Life Changes

Identify any changes you have made in your life plans, goals, work situation, etc., *since your brain injury.*	
Have you changed what college or university you attend? If yes, what did you change it from and to?	Circle: Yes / No Explain:
Have you changed your academic major? If yes, what was the change?	Circle: Yes / No Explain:
Have you changed your academic status (e.g., full time vs. part time)? If yes, what was the change?	Circle: Yes / No Explain:
Have you changed your career goal(s)? If yes, what was the change?	Circle: Yes / No Explain:
Have you changed where you live? If yes, what was the change?	Circle: Yes / No Explain:
Have you changed your current employment? If yes, what was the change?	Circle: Yes / No Explain:
Other comments:	

College Survey for Students with Concussion (CSS-C)

Name: _____ Date: _____

Interviewer: _____

I. Demographics

How old are you? _____

Sex: (Circle)   Female   Male

Are you currently enrolled in college? (Circle)   Yes   No

About how many college credits have you completed? If you attended college a long time ago, did you graduate from college? If not, how many credits did you complete? _____

_____

What years were you enrolled in college? (e.g., 2000–2004; 2006 to current) _____

_____

II. Concussion

1. Have you had a concussion? (Circle)   Yes   No

2. Was this an athletic injury?   Yes   No

3. If yes, in what sport were you injured? _____

_____

4. If no, describe how you sustained your injury. _____

_____

5. Provide the date on which you were injured: _____

_____

6. Have you been authorized to return to play your sport? If this was a long time ago, were you authorized to return to your sport? (Circle)   Yes   No   N/A

   If yes, how long ago? _____

7. Does (or did) your school have a written plan/procedure for supporting the return of student athletes to play their sport with concussion/injury? (Circle)   Yes   No   Don't know   N/A

8. Have you sustained any other type of injury (e.g., broken bone, torn tendon) since your concussion? If so, please explain. If no, respond with N/A. _____

_____

_____

(continued)

Reprinted with permission from Mary R. T. Kennedy, Gina De Salvio, and Violet Nguyen.

III. Type of Disability

What type(s) of injury and/or disability do you have, and how old were you when each occurred? Circle your answer.		
	Did you have this type of injury?	If yes, at what age?
Single concussion	Yes No	0–11 12–17 18+
Past concussions	Yes No	0–11 12–17 18+
Stroke	Yes No	0–11 12–17 18+
Brain tumor	Yes No	0–11 12–17 18+
Multiple sclerosis (MS)	Yes No	0–11 12–17 18+
Parkinson's disease	Yes No	0–11 12–17 18+
Encephalitis	Yes No	0–11 12–17 18+
Musculoskeletal injury (e.g., broken bone, torn ACL)	Yes No	0–11 12–17 18+
If musculoskeletal injury, what type?		

IV. History of Injury

Answer the following questions. Circle your answer.		
	Yes/no/don't know	If yes, approximately how long?
Did you go to the hospital for your injury?	Yes/no/don't know	Semester(s): 1 2 3 4 Day(s): 1 2 3 4 5 6 Week(s): 1 2 3 Month(s): 1 2 3 4 5 6 7 8 9 10 11 Year(s) 1 Ongoing, N/A, Other
Did you stay overnight in the hospital?	Yes/no/don't know	Semester(s): 1 2 3 4 Day(s): 1 2 3 4 5 6 Week(s): 1 2 3 Month(s): 1 2 3 4 5 6 7 8 9 10 11 Year(s) 1 Ongoing, N/A, Other
Were you unconscious or in a coma after your injury?	Yes/no/don't know	Semester(s): 1 2 3 4 Day(s): 1 2 3 4 5 6 Week(s): 1 2 3 Month(s): 1 2 3 4 5 6 7 8 9 10 11 Year(s) 1 Ongoing, N/A, Other

(continued)

	Yes/no/don't know	If yes, approximately how long?
Did you or are you now receiving any therapy or rehabilitation after your injury?	Yes/no/don't know	Semester(s): 1 2 3 4 Day(s): 1 2 3 4 5 6 Week(s): 1 2 3 Month(s): 1 2 3 4 5 6 7 8 9 10 11 Year(s) 1 Ongoing, N/A, Other
Did you take a break from work or school after your injury?	Yes/no/don't know	Semester(s): 1 2 3 4 Day(s): 1 2 3 4 5 6 Week(s): 1 2 3 Month(s): 1 2 3 4 5 6 7 8 9 10 11 Year(s) 1 Ongoing, N/A, Other
Did you get clearance to return to school?	Yes/no/don't know	Semester(s): 1 2 3 4 Day(s): 1 2 3 4 5 6 Week(s): 1 2 3 Month(s): 1 2 3 4 5 6 7 8 9 10 11 Year(s) 1 Ongoing, N/A, Other
Did you receive any specific instructions regarding returning to school?	Yes/no/don't know	Semester(s): 1 2 3 4 Day(s): 1 2 3 4 5 6 Week(s): 1 2 3 Month(s): 1 2 3 4 5 6 7 8 9 10 11 Year(s) 1 Ongoing, N/A, Other
If you received specific instructions regarding returning to school, did you follow them?	Yes/no/don't know	Semester(s): 1 2 3 4 Day(s): 1 2 3 4 5 6 Week(s): 1 2 3 Month(s): 1 2 3 4 5 6 7 8 9 10 11 Year(s) 1 Ongoing, N/A, Other
When you returned to school, did you inform your instructors that you had sustained an injury?	Yes/no/don't know	Semester(s): 1 2 3 4 Day(s): 1 2 3 4 5 6 Week(s): 1 2 3 Month(s): 1 2 3 4 5 6 7 8 9 10 11 Year(s) 1 Ongoing, N/A, Other

(continued)

If you stated Other for a length of time, explain here:

V. Effects of Injury

Indicate your biggest concerns about returning to college classes, if you have any. Circle your answer.		
Grades	Yes	No
Ability to learn	Yes	No
Amount of work	Yes	No
Headaches	Yes	No
Returning to sport	Yes	No
Fatigue	Yes	No
Other	Yes	No
If other, specify:		

Did you reduce the amount of college credits or courses you took because of your injury? (Circle)   Yes   No

Don't Know

What have been some effects of your injury? Check all that apply and indicate whether you received therapy for each effect.		
	Experienced the effect	Had therapy for this
Difficulty with academics, like studying, homework, tests		
Problems making decisions		
Difficulty with relationships, such as family		
Physical problems: arm/hands (writing, etc.)		
Mood changes and/or fluctuations		
Anger		
Physical problem: legs (walking, etc.)		
Substance/alcohol abuse		
Difficulty remembering things for school and/or at home		
Dizziness		
Headaches		
Attention problems		

(continued)

	Experienced the effect	Had therapy for this
Fatigue		
Being disorganized		
Depression or low mood		
Difficulty maintaining friendships		
Light sensitivity, especially bright lights		
Nausea		
Noise sensitivity		
Other (please specify):		

VI. Support or Therapies for Injury

Which of the following therapies/support services have you received *because* of your concussion? Circle your answer.			
Psychological counseling	None	Past (completed)	Ongoing/current
Physical therapy	None	Past (completed)	Ongoing/current
Speech or language therapy	None	Past (completed)	Ongoing/current
Occupational therapy	None	Past (completed)	Ongoing/current
Support group	None	Past (completed)	Ongoing/current
Vocational counseling	None	Past (completed)	Ongoing/current
If other, specify:			

VII. Your Student Experiences

To what extent do you agree with each of the following statements about your experience as a college student *since* your latest concussion?	Strongly disagree	Disagree	Neither agree nor disagree	Agree	Strongly agree
I forget what has been said in class.					
I get overwhelmed when studying.					
I get overwhelmed in class.					
I get nervous before tests.					
I have trouble managing my time.					
I am late to class.					
I have trouble prioritizing assignments and meeting deadlines.					

(continued)

	Strongly disagree	Disagree	Neither agree nor disagree	Agree	Strongly agree
Others do not understand my problems.					
I procrastinate on things I need to do.					
I have to review my material more than I used to.					
I don't always understand instructions for assignments.					
I have trouble reading books or magazines.					
I have trouble paying attention in class.					
I have trouble paying attention while studying.					
I have trouble doing work on a computer or other mobile devices.					
I can't study for as long as I used to prior to my injury.					
I get headaches when I read or write.					
I have fewer friends than before my injury.					
If other, specify:					
Are you interested in meeting other students with concussion? (Circle) Yes No					
Are you interested in getting help from a specialist in working with college students with concussion? (Circle) Yes No					

VIII. Your Use of Services

Since you have been in college (or when you were in college) after your concussion, did you use the following services because of challenges related to the concussion?

	Never heard of it	Heard of it, but never used	Once	Sometimes	Pretty often	All the time
Campus disability services						
Campus veterans' services						
Campus counseling services						
Campus medical services						
Campus group for students with disabilities						
State brain injury association						
State vocational rehabilitation services						
Other hospital or rehabilitation services						

(continued)

IX. Rating Services

For *any service that you have used at least once,* indicate how useful you found the service.	Completely useless	Somewhat useless	Somewhat useful	Extremely useful	N/A
Campus disability services					
Campus veterans' services					
Campus counseling services					
Campus medical services					
Campus group for students with disabilities					
State brain injury association					
State vocational rehabilitation services					
Other hospital or rehabilitation services					
Specify any other services you have received:					

X. Life Changes

Identify any changes you made in your life plans, goals, work situation, etc., because of your injury.	
Did you change the college or university you attend? If yes, what did you change it from and to?	Circle: Yes / No Explain:
Did you change your academic major? If yes, what was the change?	Circle: Yes / No Explain:
Did you change your academic status (e.g. full time vs. part time)? If yes, what was the change?	Circle: Yes / No Explain:
Did you change your career goal(s)? If yes, what was the change?	Circle: Yes / No Explain:
Did you change where you live? If yes, what was the change?	Circle: Yes / No Explain:
Did you change employment? If yes, what was the change?	Circle: Yes / No Explain:
If other, specify:	

Academic Statements from the **CSS-OD**, **CSS-BI**, and **CSS-C**, with Importance Ratings and Follow-Up Questions

Instructions

1. Record students' responses from the academic challenges listed on Forms 5.4, 5, 5, and 5.6.

2. Ask students to rate the importance of each one, using the scale of 1 to 5 below.

   1 = not important at all   4 = important

   2 = not important   5 = very important

   3 = uncertain how important this is

3. Follow up with probing interview questions that give students the opportunity to describe what happens, if they are using strategies, and if they think their strategies are working.

4. Consider the challenges with which the students agreed (ratings of 4 or 5); then consider the importance of the challenges to the students (ratings of 4 or 5). Students with high ratings—that is, those who agree to having particular challenges—should be asked to explore their importance ratings in more detail and if highly important to the student, coaches and students can target these areas immediately (i.e., these become immediate proximal goals).

5. Have students highlight the challenges by category from Forms 5.4, 5.5, and 5.6. Use this organization to discuss the specific challenges and the domains to be addressed.

6. This form can be used at the beginning of the semester or year and again at the end of the semester or year.

   a. A comparison of ratings over time can be used as evidence that students' awareness has improved.

   b. When students report using more strategies and different strategies, this can be interrupted as deeper awareness when corroborated with other positive outcomes (e.g., being able to study for longer periods of time or improved grades on exams).

7. *Agreement* ratings are 1 (strongly disagree) to 5 (strongly agree). *Importance* ratings are 1 (very unimportant) to 5 (very important). *Categories* are learning and studying (LS), managing and organizing (MO), social advocacy (SA), and stress (ST).

(continued)

Academic Statements from the CSS-OD

Statement	Agreement rating (1 to 5)	Importance rating (1 to 5)	Category MO, LS, SA, ST	Interview questions: What do you do when this happens? Are there things you've tried in order to change this? Do you use any strategies?
I procrastinate on things I need to do.			MO	
I get overwhelmed when studying.			LS	
I get overwhelmed in class.			NS, LS	
I get nervous before tests.			NS	
I have trouble managing my time.			MO	
I am late to class.			MO	
I have trouble meeting deadlines.			MO	
I have trouble prioritizing assignments.			MO	
Others do not understand my problems.			SA	
I forget what has been said in class.			LS	
I have fewer friends than I thought I would have.			SA	

(continued)

144

Academic Statements from the CSS-OD *(page 2 of 2)*

Statement	Agreement rating (1 to 5)	Importance rating (1 to 5)	Category MO, LS, SA, ST	Interview questions: What do you do when this happens? Are there things you've tried in order to change this? Do you use any strategies?
I don't always understand instructions for assignments.			LS	
I get distracted while studying.			LS	
I have to review material more than I thought I would.			LS	
I get distracted in class.			LS	
I don't know how to start large projects.			MO	
The assignments I turn in are messy or disorganized.			MO	
I get impatient when working in groups.			NS	
I have trouble understanding what I read in textbooks.			LS	
I get frustrated easily.			NS	
I forget what friends or family tell me.			LS	
I tend to say what I think regardless of the situation.			NS, SA	
I have trouble following through on things I say I will do.			MO	
I don't socialize with friends as much as I would like.			SA	

145

Academic Statements from the CSS-BI

Statement	Agreement rating (1 to 5)	Importance rating (1 to 5)	Category MO, LS, SA, ST	Interview questions: What do you do when this happens? Are there things you've tried in order to change this? Do you use any strategies?
I have to review material more than I used to.			LS	
I have fewer friends than before.			SA	
I have trouble prioritizing assignments and meeting deadlines.			MO, LS	
I procrastinate on things I need to do.			MO	
I have trouble managing my time.			MO	
I am late to class.			MO	
I have trouble paying attention in class or while studying			MO, LS	
I don't always understand instructions for assignments.			LS	
Others do not understand my problems.			SA	
I get overwhelmed when studying.			NS	
I get nervous before tests.			NS	
I get overwhelmed in class.			LS	
I forget what has been said in class.			LS	

146

Academic Statements from the CSS-C

Statement	Agreement rating (1 to 5)	Importance rating (1 to 5)	Category MO, LS, SA, ST	Interview questions: What do you do when this happens? Are there things you've tried in order to change this? Do you use any strategies?
I have to review material more than I used to.			LS	
I have fewer friends than before.			SA	
I have trouble prioritizing assignments and meeting deadlines.			MO, LS	
I procrastinate on things I need to do.			MO	
I have trouble doing work on a computer or other mobile devices.			LS	
I have trouble managing my time.			MO	
I am late to class.			MO	
I have trouble paying attention in class.			MO, LS	
I don't always understand instructions for assignments.			LS	
Others do not understand my problems.			SA	
I get overwhelmed when studying.			ST	

(continued)

Academic Statements from the CSS-C *(page 2 of 2)*

Statement	Agreement rating (1 to 5)	Importance rating (1 to 5)	Category MO, LS, SA, ST	Interview questions: What do you do when this happens? Are there things you've tried in order to change this? Do you use any strategies?
I have trouble reading books or magazines.			ST	
I can't study for as long as I used to prior to my injury.			ST	
I get nervous before tests.			ST	
I get overwhelmed in class.			LS	
I forget what has been said in class.			LS	
I have trouble paying attention while studying.			MO, LS	

FORM 5.8

Interpreting **Abilities** and **Disabilities**

Name: _____   Date: _____

I am able to:

Examples of this are:

1. _____

    1. _____

    2. _____

    3. _____

2. _____

    1. _____

    2. _____

    3. _____

3. _____

    1. _____

    2. _____

    3. _____

4. _____

    1. _____

    2. _____

    3. _____

(continued)

Interpreting Abilities and Disabilities *(page 2 of 2)*

I have difficulty with:

1. _____

2. _____

3. _____

4. _____

Examples of this are:

1. _____

2. _____

3. _____

1. _____

2. _____

3. _____

1. _____

2. _____

3. _____

1. _____

2. _____

3. _____

Templates for Goal Attainment Scaling

Instructions

1. Collaborate with students to create SMARTER goals using these templates.

2. Discuss how the steps involved toward reaching the target goal will show that performance has improved or declined.

   Note that the four forms have different starting points and target points.

   Two forms use ratings of +2 to –2.

   Two forms use ratings of +1 to +5.

   Two forms designate a one-point difference between the starting point and target.

   Two forms designate a two-point difference between the starting point and target.

3. To start, let the student choose the template. As you develop the goal, the template may change depending on the number of steps that are created to reach the goal.

(continued)

Goal:		
	2	
Target	1	
Starting Point	0	
	−1	
	−2	
Notes		

(continued)

Goal:		
	2	
Target	1	
	0	
Starting Point	−1	
	−2	
Notes		

(continued)

Goal:		
	5	
Target	4	
Starting Point	3	
	2	
	1	
Notes		

(continued)

Goal:		
	5	
Target	4	
	3	
Starting Point	2	
	1	
Notes		

A List of Goals by Immediacy, Ranging from **Weeks** to **Years**

Goal	This week	Week to month	Current semester	Academic year	2+ years	Notes
	Now		Proximal		Distal	

Mapping Proximal and Distal Goals onto a Plan by Immediacy of Need

Immediate: *Today to This Week*

-
-
-

Proximal: *Next Week to Month*

-
-
-

Proximal: *During Semester*

-
-
-

(continued)

Proximal: *During Academic Year*

-
-
-

Distal: *During 2 Years*

-
-
-

Distal: *Long-Term Goals*

-
-
-

CHAPTER 6

Coaching Self-Management and Self-Learning

Goals–Strategies–Act–Adjust

with Katy H. O'Brien

We now know that the primary challenges of students with deficits in executive function fall into three broad categories: self-learning, self-management, and self-advocacy. In this chapter, we dig deeper into the first two of these, and in Chapter 7, we talk more about self-advocacy. Here we discuss how coaches can map an intervention program addressing self-learning and self-management onto the Goals–Strategies–Act–Adjust (GSAA) framework first described in Chapter 4. Specifically, we revisit *Goal* setting in regard to these specific domains, then turn to *Strategy* selection, followed by a discussion of supporting students as they *Act* on those strategies. Finally, we discuss the steps involved in having students assess their own performance and *Adjust* as necessary. Along the way, this chapter also addresses challenges specific to these domains, and provides examples of low- and high-technology strategies.

Why are we combining two of these rather large domains together in this chapter? Essentially because, the more time we spent with students with executive function problems, the clearer it became that these two domains are intertwined so that addressing each in isolation provided an incomplete coaching approach. Consider this: On the CSS-BI, almost all students reported a need to spend more time reviewing material. Although students spend this extra time reviewing so

Katy H. O'Brien, PhD, CCC-SLP, Department of Communication Sciences and Special Education, University of Georgia, Athens, Georgia

that they can *learn* what is needed for class, students must also be able to *plan* for this extra study time in order to be effective learners. Therefore, if we were to spend this chapter discussing only the approach to managing studying and learning, it would be incomplete because students must also fit those strategies into their tight schedules. Therefore, coaching students to regulate their learning involves coaching them to also manage their time and set priorities.

Discussing these two domains in isolation also runs the risk of oversimplifying the issues that students may be dealing with. Coaches can make the implementation phase more effective by acknowledging that in asking students to use new strategies, they are also asking them to devote more time to planning how to complete their work. Initially, deploying new strategies consistently can be laborious and time-consuming. Remember that the student is committing time and effort when adding a new strategy. However, eventually, those strategies that are retained should become more fluid and result in a reasonable trade-off of effort and gain. When coaches acknowledge the complexity of these two domains and discuss these potential barriers up front, they validate the challenge for the student and present a more realistic picture of the implementation phase. Together, student and coach can then manage these challenges as part of the intervention plan.

Of course, oftentimes ineffective strategies that students are using may be inefficient as well. Students entering college with executive function problems have grown accustomed to using certain strategies that helped them succeed in high school. Students with an ABI, on the other hand, will rely on strategies used prior to their injury, which may not work with their new disability. Therefore, it can be helpful for the student and coach to describe how swapping a "bad" strategy for a "good" one will eventually lead to improved efficiency and performance. Take, as an example, cramming before exams, which is ubiquitous and, on its face, feels effective and efficient. Students may think that cramming will ensure that the material feels "fresh" during test taking. In fact, this kind of studying produces an illusion of learning (Koriat & Bjork, 2005). Limited retrieval practice means that students will be unlikely to recall studied information and that the strength of that stored information will rapidly deteriorate. It is also particularly problematic if the course material or future exams rely on previous knowledge. This poor study habit sets students up for failure for the rest of the semester and increases the amount of future time that will have to be spent relearning old material. Instead, having a student plan his or her studying over a period of time leading up to an exam will be more time-consuming on the front end, but will reap the benefits of increased efficiency and performance at the semester progresses. Besides improved learning, engaging in regular studying also reduces the feeling of being stressed (Pham & Taylor, 1999).

Metacognitive beliefs and ongoing monitoring often operate independently of one another; a student may believe that a strategy will be successful, but not observe the evidence of failure as an indicator that the strategy was ineffective (Dunning, Johnson, Ehrlinger, & Kruger, 2005; Kennedy & Coelho, 2005). In this situation, coaches can support students in being careful observers of their own behavior and in adjusting strategies in response to outcomes.

Bjork and Bjork (2011) reviewed a number of learning effects that appear counterintuitive on the surface, particularly to students unaccustomed to considering the distinction between short-term and long-term learning. Although students often strive for studying to feel easier, rather than harder, the authors propose four "desirable" difficulties to foster learning and recall. In addition to the importance of distributed over massed (i.e., cramming) practice, the literature reviewed by these authors indicates that students should interleave rather than block their studying. Students may be tempted to study all of their chemistry material, followed by all of their Spanish. Interleaving involves studying one topic or area, followed by a different topic, and so on during a single session. It allows for forgetting when concentrating on the alternate topic, increasing retrieval strength with subsequent exposure.

Third, students may prefer having study guides provided by professors prior to exams, but the generation effect (as described in Chapter 4) shows that a student is more likely to recall material that was sought out, created, and actively recalled, rather than simply handed to them. When students create their own study guides, they are activating a broader network of to-be-recalled information and, therefore, are processing the information on a deeper level than "reviewing" what someone else has given them. Finally, students often study by reviewing material repeatedly, but exams require not just that information be stored, but that the student be able to retrieve it rapidly and accurately. Few students take the time to practice this latter skill, even though one of the most powerful tools of learning is testing itself. When self-quizzing, students have the opportunity to practice retrieval, but more important, to activate the metacognitive system by observing their performance. Coaches can educate students about such learning effects, but wield a more powerful tool when they have students observe the successes of such strategy adjustments themselves. These evidence-based ways of making studying "harder" map nicely onto the characteristics of dynamic coaching identified in Chapter 4.

The metacognitive aspect of learning cannot be overemphasized. Kennedy and colleagues have shown that adults with TBI can effectively monitor their memory and learning under certain conditions. For example, adults with TBI tend to be very accurate at knowing whether or not an item had been completely forgotten or accurately remembered, but were overly confident when they were unsure (Kennedy, 2001; Kennedy & Yorkston, 2000). In contrast, adults without TBI were underconfident, thinking information had been forgotten when it was not. In a follow-up study linking this self-monitoring with strategy decisions, adults with TBI were more accurate than a computer algorithm at selecting items they should restudy

(Kennedy, Carney, & Peters, 2003). This finding underscores the importance of supporting self-regulation in learners. Learners have idiosyncratic knowledge about their own cognitive processes and their own personal knowledge that allows them to best select strategies. However, these learners often need targeted instruction to monitor their performance and reestablish an effective self-regulation loop. This chapter aims to provide a coach with the steps to do just that.

GOAL SETTING IN SELF-LEARNING

After the college student survey or questionnaire, the semistructured interview, and reviewing a student's history have been completed, the time has come for the student and coach to meet and figure out what the student's needs are with respect to studying and learning. The following questions about the student's courseload can set the stage for the student to consider the context of his or her learning and studying needs:

- What classes are you taking?
- How many hours of credit are given for each class?
- How often do classes meet?
- How long are your classes?
- What are the course requirements?
  - How many exams are given? What is the format (multiple choice, essay, online, etc.)?
  - Are there papers or presentations?
- What are the reading expectations?
- Is there any group work?

The type of classes the student is taking during a semester will generate other questions. From this starting point, though, the coach should steer the conversation toward the student's anticipated needs. The CSS-BI gives a general overview of student academic experiences, but now the coach and student can determine how those challenges may play out in this particular semester with these particular classes.

Goals are self-identified with the support of the coach. Students tend to describe their needs broadly, so that the role of the coach often involves questioning students to define how they view that goal. In Chapter 5, Table 5.3 gave examples of how self-regulation and performance goals are related; here Table 6.1 lists examples of the kinds of statements students may make about their goals, and how

TABLE 6.1. Sample Goal Development for Studying and Learning

Student goal	Coaching follow-up	Example self-regulation goal	Example performance goal
"I want to do well this semester."	"Tell me a little more about that. What do your grades look like now? What does doing well mean for you? Do you have a particular grade in mind? How about for different classes—do you have different expectations of what doing well might look like in different classes?"	The student will monitor grades across the course of the semester, using a self-generated spreadsheet based on course syllabi.	The student will earn an overall GPA of 3.5. The student will earn a grade of B in Organic Chemistry. The student will earn a grade of A in the English seminar.
"I've got to get better at taking tests. I never feel like I know enough."	"Tell me what kinds of tests are challenging for you—for example, are essays or multiple choice more challenging?" "What kinds of things are you doing to help your test taking now?" "What do you think would be most helpful in feeling like you know the material?"	The student will identify four strategies to use when studying for exams, then adjust strategies based on exam performance.	The student will earn a grade of at least a C on all exams this semester in Statistics.
"I have to read and reread. I'd really like to be able to remember what I read better."	"What kind of reading do you have to do this semester?" "Which classes concern you most?"	The student will self-cue to use keyword strategy by explicitly monitoring reading recall, asking himself at the end of each page, "What did I just read?"	The student will recall main details from chapters read in English Literature class with 90% accuracy.
"I have lots of vocabulary for Spanish that I need to learn. It's hard to get it to stick."	"What strategies have you been using? Are any of them working?"	The student will use flashcards to self-assess learning, making stacks of "correct," "almost," and "missed," to guide studying items most needed.	The student will recall 90% of vocabulary words studied each week.

questioning them using the principles from MI can lead to goals that are more defined and student centered. Looking at these goals, it may already become clear that we will also need to plan when and how the student will meet these goals. Let's talk more about self-management goals and then return to this table to see how goals might align for these two domains.

One example of a studying and learning goal created with coaching support is that of a student with significant memory impairments who was having difficulty remembering what he was reading in a novel assigned for class. He had used a reading journal in a previous course and selected that strategy to use again to support his recall. For each chapter he read, he would write a brief summary of key events and characters so that he could quickly scan the journal rather than rereading many pages of text. With his coach, this student developed a goal attainment scale (GAS) as described in Chapter 5. Figure 6.1 is the scaled goal that they created together.

Another student had mild difficulty with word-finding, as well as the executive function problems of planning and staying organized, so that writing essays was daunting. The student wanted to do well on her papers and set a performance goal of earning an A on all written essays. The coach and student developed a paired self-regulation goal to learn how she writes papers best. Together, they set up an iterative process mirroring that of the GSAA cycle to support each step of writing a paper, from brainstorming, to generating an outline, to producing a thesis statement, to writing a draft, then editing and continuing to write to produce a quality document, as listed in Figure 6.2 (using the step-by-step approach shown in Form 4.6, Action Planning). For each step, the student had specific action plans, and then reported back to the coach whether the strategy was successful. Together, they reviewed the products of each step to determine what could be more effective for the next step or for the next paper. The coach used MI during weekly sessions, guiding the student toward self-evaluation rather than providing directive

Self-Learning Goal: Reading Journal		
	5	Writing summaries of chapters read for all chapters. Notes effectively trigger specific and consistent recall of events and characters. Scanning of the book is limited to specific scenarios, such as using quotes for an essay. Notes are well elaborated and allow for integration of ideas across the narrative. *(Notes trigger recall **all** of the time.)*
	4	Writing summaries of chapters read for all chapters. The effectiveness of notes in triggering recall is fairly consistent, so that only minimal scanning of the book is needed to recall details. Notes are well elaborated. *(Notes trigger recall **almost all** of the time.)*
Target	3	Writing summaries of chapters read for most chapters, so that most chapters have notes, but some still may not. Alternatively, all chapters have notes, but the effectiveness of notes in triggering recall is inconsistent. Some book scanning still occurs, rather than relying on summaries alone. *(Notes trigger recall **most** of the time.)*
Starting Point	2	Writing summaries of chapters read only occasionally, so that some chapters have notes, but others may have none at all. The effectiveness of notes in triggering recall is inconsistent. You are more often scanning the book rather than relying on summaries. *(Notes trigger recall **sometimes**.)*
	1	Writing summaries of chapters read only rarely or not at all.

FIGURE 6.1. Sample scaled self-learning goal using GAS.

Goal: *Earn a grade of A on all written papers/Learn how I write papers best.*

Steps in my plan	Done (✓)	E = easy; R = routine; H = hard	
		Will be . . .	Was
1. *Brainstorm: work with coach and independently to generate at least five arguments and supporting ideas.* Due date: *1 week*	✓	*H*	*R*
2. *Generate an outline: include introduction, background, thesis, organized arguments in a logical order, conclusion.* Due date: *2 weeks*	✓	*R*	*H*
3. *Write a thesis statement: use thesis statement handout from class, meet with teaching assistant.* Due date: *3 weeks*	✓	*H*	*R*
4. *Write a first draft: all components of outline, but conclusion can be preliminary, write 1 hour a day in library after class Mondays, Wednesdays, Fridays, then 2 hours on Saturdays; writing time can include research time.* Due date: *5 weeks*	✓	*H*	*R*
5. *Edit draft: swap with peer for general feedback, read paper aloud at home in room, spend writing time from previous schedule, meet with teaching assistant again.* Due date: *6 weeks*	✓	*E*	*H*
6. *Write second draft, cycle back as needed: continue steps from 4 and 5, discuss with coach as needed.* Due date: *7 to 8 weeks*	✓	*H*	*R*

How well did this plan work? Did you accomplish your goal?

It was definitely helpful. I feel a lot more confident in my writing, even though the time commitment was really big. I had to think about this really far in advance, but it left me time to contact the teaching assistant when I was confused. I could also take my thesis and outline to her to make sure I was on track, so that made it very worthwhile to plan that far ahead. I got an A, so that was great too. Hopefully next time I can use this plan to write another quality paper.

- **Were all of the steps needed?**

   All of the steps were definitely needed.

- **Were there additional steps that you did not anticipate? Which ones?**

   I ended up editing a lot along the way though. Even my outline got edited quite a bit; I didn't expect that going into this. Now I know to allow time for that, and that it's OK if I change where I was going with the paper if it still works.

(continued)

FIGURE 6.2. Action-Planning Form (Form 4.6) for a student with memory impairments.

- **Were the steps as hard as you anticipated?**

  Some were easier, like brainstorming, although we worked together on that. Things like the thesis were easier because I had plenty of time—I didn't have to just rush something that wasn't really thought out and then didn't really work for the paper. Editing was a lot harder than I thought. I just wanted to be done sometimes, or my attention would drift. But it definitely made my paper better to keep working on it.

- **Would you do anything differently next time?**

  We worked together on a lot of it, so mostly I want to practice doing all of this myself next time. I'm still a little worried about getting started, coming up with ideas to get me going. Maybe even if I don't have a coach, next time I can meet with classmates to discuss our ideas.

FIGURE 6.2. *(continued)*

feedback. The process therefore taught the student not just the steps involved in writing a paper as listed in Figure 6.2, but more important, how to evaluate her own writing so that she could make adjustments as necessary. The paired goal no doubt allowed her to write better papers during the semester in which she received coaching support, but the self-regulation goal set her up not only to achieve that goal, but also to continue to perform well on subsequent writing assignments.

From this example, two points should be emphasized. First, despite the student's word-finding impairment, it was coaching support in organizing and structuring her papers that was most helpful for this student to be successful. As described in earlier chapters, remediating executive function problems is critical to managing other co-occurring cognitive impairments. Having a clear plan and discrete steps in place freed up cognitive resources or "space" for her to use her word-finding strategies when writing. Second, developing the plan for writing a paper again took more time initially and required the student to start this project weeks ahead of time. Even though writing papers falls into the domain of self-learning, the planning and scheduling necessary to manage a studying and learning deficit in this area required concomitant support in the domain of self-management.

GOAL SETTING IN SELF-MANAGEMENT

Students who have some college experience tend to have a better grasp on the importance of this domain to their academic success. Those who are entering as freshman and may have had supports in place during high school (not to mention highly routinized schedules) may have a harder time predicting the role that time management will have in supporting their success, or underlying their failures, in the other domains. In fact, we have found that regardless of a student's profile, all students benefit from organizing and managing their time well.

Student time-management needs tend to fall into a few categories. Students need to manage their time effectively in order to complete:

- Daily routines
- Short-term assignments
- Long-term assignments that must be completed over a period of time (i.e., larger projects, presentations, labwork)
- Studying
- Extracurricular activities

Of course, this list is not exhaustive. Students are also frequently scheduling other meetings and needs into their time. Note that the categories are listed from the most scheduled to the least, so that routine activities, such as classes, are highly predictable and their times can be entered with confidence into a student planner or calendar far in advance. Although students must initially adapt to changes in schedules at the beginning of each semester, they typically are able to establish routines of when and where they need to be fairly quickly. The same is true of specific short-term assignments. The syllabus likely provides specifics about what is due when; however, students must schedule the time in their week to complete the assignment. Long-term assignments are less structured; students must not only plan ahead to complete these assignments, but do so over an extended period of time, setting subgoals to ensure timely completion. Studying is even less structured; students might know when there are upcoming exams, but must plan time independently to ensure that they are reviewing material frequently. Finding time for extracurricular activities poses yet another challenge for students, and we discuss that in greater depth in Chapter 7.

These tasks are increasingly difficult for students with executive function problems, as evidenced from our own coaching experiences and research findings (e.g., Kennedy & Krause, 2011; Kennedy et al., 2014). We found that students did not agree that they are late to class, but did believe that they had difficulty with procrastination, prioritizing, and managing their time and acknowledged that arriving to appointments on time is a prerequisite skill for college and "the least they could do" to support their learning. Other students explicitly linked the feeling of being overwhelmed with poor time management, so that having to complete work quickly was stressful and contributed to poor performance. Virtually all students agreed that they needed to review material more, which is likely related to the ubiquity of reported time-management needs. Students also reported that when they allowed themselves an appropriate amount of time to complete their work, stress levels decreased and the quality of their work improved.

Students tend to need more coaching support in identifying time-management goals. Probing for strategies already in place is a good place to start. Many students use a planner system, but these systems vary. Despite the temptation to assume that students will prefer to use a high-tech option like a smartphone, many students still rely on printed schedules or hard copies of planners, particularly those provided by colleges that include school holidays and other important dates (drop/add dates, tuition billing cycles, final exams, and graduation). Coaches should ask students about their preferences. Students typically add class meeting times to the calendar at the beginning of the semester but may use a different system to keep track of assignments or none at all for long-term projects or study time.

Here is an example of a student using different types of time-management systems. This student had struggled to use his planner, only intermittently entering items or accessing it. The coach began to probe again for how this student was managing his schedule if the planner was no longer being used. The student then produced a folded piece of paper from the first week of the semester with color-coded blocks of his weekly schedule. He reported making it at the beginning of the semester, and now he had a habit of keeping it in his pocket as a reminder. Because it was a printed copy, coaching focused on developing this strategy to manage other aspects of his weekly schedule. Each Sunday, he would print out a new schedule and fill in specific information for the week, then continue carrying it in his pocket until the next week, when it would be updated.

Another student needed to develop a system from scratch. She had been unable to use a store-bought planner because she needed more structure than a generic planner could provide. She had been struggling in her courses, primarily because assignments were not being turned in on time or were not completed correctly. In fact, it was unclear if the student was actually struggling with self-learning because her self-management problems were overshadowing her ability to demonstrate her knowledge. With support from her coach, she identified items that she needed to add to the planner in order for her to keep up with her assignments and daily schedule. The planner went through a series of piloting and revision cycles (again mirroring that of GSAA), but settled on a printed system that had checkboxes for her to select which courses had new assignments, and that featured columns for notes, page numbers or where to find the assignment, due dates, and every student's favorite—a box showing the task had been completed.

Table 6.2 shows how what a student might describe as a problem or goal can be developed into paired performance and self-regulation goals. Note that the coach probes for specificity, setting priorities, current strategies, and how a student visualizes success. For example, the student stated that she or he needs to allow more time to get things done. Upon further questioning, the student realized that both studying and not keeping up with weekly assignments seemed to fall through the cracks. The student can then set a goal on making sure time is scheduled for these

TABLE 6.2. Sample Goal Development for Time Management

Student goal	Coaching follow-up	Example self-regulation goal	Example performance goal
"I need to keep track of my assignments better."	"Tell me a little more about that. What do you do to keep up with your assignments now? What would it look like for you to keep track of your assignments perfectly?"	Student will monitor accuracy of planner by checking syllabus at least once a week. Student will monitor assignment tracking by asking himself before leaving class each day, did I add all new assignments to my planner?	Student will enter all assignments into planner. Student will create a weekly to-do list using the syllabus and class notes. Student will create a planner that reflects the needs of class assignments.
"It feels like I am always a day or week behind and scrambling to catch up. I'd like to feel like I have my schedule under control."	"Tell me what kinds of assignments are challenging for you—for example, just the number of assignments you have to do, or bigger projects, exams?" "What kinds of things are you doing to keep track of assignments now?" "What do you think would be most helpful in feeling like your schedule is under control?"	Student will identify three strategies to use when scheduling long-term assignments. Student will schedule time for bigger assignments explicitly in planner, specifying the goal, time, and place (e.g., write outline for final paper from 11:00 to 1:00 on Tuesday at library). Student will create a GAS self-rating scale of procrastination and "hurriedness" of projects.	Student will submit all assignments on time. Student will minimize procrastination and feeling of being rushed, as measured by self-rating GAS scale scores of 4 or better.
"I need to give myself enough time to get things done."	"What kinds of things are you not giving yourself enough time for? Which aspects of your schedule or assignments concern you most?"	Student will use plan–do–review to make predictions about time needed for completion of school tasks, then compare predictions with actual time.	Student will schedule studying into weekly calendar, allowing 1.5 times current estimates.
"I've got a class that requires me to work in a group the whole semester, so I've got to find time to meet with the members."	"What kind of work will you be doing with your group? Will you be meeting in person, or will some of these meetings be virtual? Do you know the people in your group?"	Student will monitor how frequently s/he reschedules or cancels group meetings to ensure that s/he is contributing to group functioning.	Student will prioritize group meetings, flexibly rescheduling personal tasks if the group is not available at other times, so that greater than 90% of meetings occur as scheduled. Student will install Skype (or Google Hangouts, etc.) to allow for virtual meetings with group.

less-structured academic needs and can learn to self-regulate his or her scheduling by becoming more accurate at knowing how much time is actually needed.

As a final thought on goal setting in these two domains, note that pairing performance and self-regulation goals acknowledges the role that self-regulation plays in meeting performance goals. Self-regulation goals are the tools that students use to meet performance goals. Looking back across the rows in Tables 6.1 and 6.2, the self-regulation goals are not necessarily exhaustive examples of how performance goals can be met, but instead indicate particular areas of need that students selected to address in order to achieve desired performance. This is yet another benefit of the self-regulation approach—it focuses the student on the process required to meet a goal, rather than fixating on the goal itself. Research in academic settings has shown that college students are more likely to succeed when carefully considering the steps involved in achieving success rather than focusing on the outcome alone. Students who focus solely on the outcome tend to lower their original goals rather than to change behaviors to meet them, such as deciding to shoot for a B instead of an A on an exam (Pham & Taylor, 1999; Taylor, 2011).

STRATEGIZING FOR SELF-LEARNING

Table 6.3 is a list of learning and study strategies and memory techniques that include some aspect of self-regulation (e.g., predicting, self-quizzing, reflection) and are recommended based on high levels of research evidence (Dunlosky, Hertzog, Kennedy, & Theide, 2005; O'Neil-Pirozzi, Kennedy, & Sohlberg, 2016; Sohlberg & Turkstra, 2011; Velikonja et al., 2014). We have found these strategies useful when working with students with executive function problems who also have difficulty with paying attention and remembering material for class. What's more, each of these strategies involves several steps that force students to study at a deeper level of processing than highlighting and repeating. More passive study techniques do little to help students with learning difficulties remember what they've studied, and also leave them with only a feeling of familiarity with the material or the illusion of knowing it.

These learning and study strategies can help students get off to a good start, particularly at the onset of coaching when students may feel less sure about how to approach their learning needs. There are also a multitude of study strategies offered online, and often colleges and universities have their own study guides provided as part of freshman orientation or tutoring programs. Self-regulation coaching adds value to these resources by teaching students (1) how to select strategies that are best for their needs, (2) how to implement those strategies in a manner that can be sustained, (3) and how to modify the strategy based on their individualized needs.

TABLE 6.3. Studying, Learning, and Memory Techniques That Include Aspects of Self-Regulation

Strategy	Description
Visual imagery	Using mental visualizing to link the to-be-remembered information or locations to images.
Elaborative encoding (verbal and/or written)	Associating information through images, words, and items to be remembered.
Story method	Creating a story that connects related bits of pieces of information to be remembered.
Retrieval techniques (e.g., mental retracing, alphabetical searching, delayed self-quizzing)	Systematically recalling, retrieving, and pulling out of memory previously studied information to trigger target information, and then restudying what was not recalled.
Preview–Question–Review–Study–Test (PQRST)	A study method in which students preview material to be read/studied/learned, review questions/purpose of the material while studying, read/review the material and self-reflect, followed by a self-test or quiz.
Keyword approach to note taking	A note-taking technique while reading, reviewing notes, and listening to a lecture. Students write important content words that will likely trigger recall for the material to be learned.

Many students use flashcards as a tool to learn rote information. If students are simply reading one side of the card, then quickly checking the answer on the back, this is unlikely to be an effective strategy. However, small adjustments to this existing routine can make the strategy more effective. For one student, this meant making a judgment as to whether the information on a card had been well learned, familiar, or not yet learned. The student made three groups, one for each category. The student then spent more time on the familiar and not-yet-learned stacks, slowly moving each into the well-learned pile. This adjustment allowed the student to focus his efforts on items that most needed it, while interleaving practice with the other items. The student was also explicitly practicing self-assessment with each item. Another student used flashcards to learn new vocabulary for an anatomy and biology class. Taking both classes in the same semester, he would sometimes confuse the two lists of words. He decided to select a strategy of using different-colored notecards and pens, so that he learned to associate certain colors with each set of words. For a third student, placing more emphasis on making the flashcards for her Spanish class allowed for richer encoding of the material. The student would write the word on the front of the card and add a small picture. On the back, she would write the translation and use it in a sentence. When reviewing the cards, she used the same routine of deciding whether words had been well learned, so that strategies were combined to make for a successful studying routine.

Adjusting existing routines to be more effective can be a powerful tool because the student already has a framework for how a strategy works and how much time is required. In other cases, entirely new strategies will have to be developed. Consider the student who had learned to take notes using a smartpen that records the lecture while taking notes on special paper. When reviewing lectures, students click on their notes to replay that audio portion of the lecture. The student used the Strategy Usefulness and Next Steps form (Form 4.5) to report that he felt that he was taking too many notes and not paying enough attention to the lecture. He found that when he reviewed the audio with his notes, he just listened to that part of the lecture again. Given the level of his memory impairment, it was clear that he could benefit from processing the information at a deeper level later when listening and reviewing his notes. Together, the coach and student changed the note-taking process without drastically changing how he used the smartpen. Here is what he did:

1. He drew a vertical line down the middle of the page before taking notes.
2. He took notes in sentence fragments, rather than in complete sentences. Notes were written on the left side of the page only.
3. While reviewing notes and listening to the lecture, he took additional notes on the right side of the page to fill in what he had missed.

These note-taking changes not only allowed him to process the information at a deeper level while reviewing, but also allowed him to listen more carefully and to take fewer notes during the lecture. Furthermore, by tracking the amount of notes on the right side of the page, he could see that for some lectures, additional notes were seldom needed. With practice, his note-taking-while-listening improved, as demonstrated by fewer and fewer additional notes on the right side of the page.

Students are often managing attention deficits both in the classroom and while studying. There are again a wide variety of available resources or tools for attention management. Many of our students reported successfully using strategies that fall into a category known as "environmental structuring" (O'Brien et al., 2017; Zimmerman & Martinez-Pons, 1986), in which they essentially manipulate their environment to maximize their attention. In the classroom, many students found that sitting at the front of the class helped them focus their attention on the teacher and avoid the distractions of their classmates (and their often off-topic computer use). One student also reported needing to have a clock visible so that she keep could pace herself, breaking the class into 10-minute segments. Study time solutions varied widely, and reflect the idiosyncrasies of learners. Some students preferred studying at home; others needed to go somewhere very quiet, like the library. Others needed a balance of the two, choosing a favorite coffee shop to surround themselves with other people working, but with a low hum of activity to keep them engaged in their work. Coaches should consider such structuring when students report attention deficits and specifically ask students to describe their current concerns and routines.

Other students need more specific strategies to manage attention problems. During class, a student was having difficulty keeping pace with the instructor when taking notes. As part of his accommodations, a note taker was arranged to provide notes so that he could focus his efforts on attending to the lecture and not his frustrations with his slow writing. The professor encouraged him to listen only, rather than multitasking by taking some notes. However, the student quickly found that when he was only sitting in class, it was hard to stay engaged with the lecture. His attention would drift easily, and he was recalling less and less, even with the better notes that he received from his peer. The student decided to bridge the two extremes and take minimal notes as a way to continue to remind himself of the key points in the lecture and to feel that he was a part of the class. His recall continued to be supported by the notes provided to him, but his attention was managed by using note taking to engage himself in the class.

Another student struggled to concentrate while reading. A previous therapist had suggested that she spend 20 minutes reading, then 20 minutes doing something else. When she met with us for coaching, she immediately reported feeling frustrated that she had not been able to get this strategy to work for her. Spending 20 minutes on another activity was getting her even more distracted, so that it was hard for her to return to work. While it may seem logical that this strategy needed to be adjusted, this student's executive function problems reinforced her rigidity in using a strategy that had been suggested by a professional. Rather than assuming there was something wrong with the strategy, she blamed herself for the failure and her attention problem. Later in the chapter, we cover strategy adjustment in greater detail, but we note here that the strength of teaching self-regulation rather than strategies is that students can also *learn to correctly situate their difficulties as problems to be solved rather than as character flaws*. With the help of the coach, this student decided to read for 20 minutes, decrease her "break" time to 2 minutes, followed by reading for a different class for 20 minutes, followed by a 5-minute break before repeating the cycle. After 1 week, she reported increased satisfaction with the strategy and her reading recall.

In all of these examples, the focus was not on strategy instruction, although that may need to occur, especially for students with memory and learning impairments. But here, the self-regulation approach is teaching students how to monitor, select, and deploy appropriate strategies and modify them if needed to continually improve performance. Coaches may provide strategy options, but whenever possible should allow students to develop or modify strategies to best meet their needs, personal preferences, and situational constraints. As recommended in an extensive review of the attention therapy literature, Ponsford and colleagues (2014) concluded that research evidence indeed supports using metacognitive training, and even behavioral therapy, for attention deficits when the intent is to improve practical everyday activities.

STRATEGIZING FOR SELF-MANAGEMENT

As goals become more specific and are clearly defined as related to either performance or self-regulation, they can then be used to direct the intervention approach. Using Form 5.11, the coach and student can prioritize goals by immediacy of need in order to make a plan. If coaches did not explicitly question students about current strategies during goal development, this is also a good time to review what systems the student has in place. In setting goals for the plan, the coach can ask students what strategies are being used and to what degree those strategies have been effective.

At this point, the coach should return to Figure 4.2 to explain the cycle of goal setting, strategizing, creating an action plan, and adjusting that will be used throughout the coaching program. The coach can explain that for each goal, he or she will support the student in developing strategies to address that need, then the student will monitor whether that strategy is helping him or her to get closer to that goal. Together, they can discuss the kind of adjustments that might need to be made to continue realizing the goal. Such a conversation might go as follows:

COACH: So you want to better manage large projects so that all components are turned in on time and are of sufficient quality to earn at least a grade of B. And that you want to feel positive, rather than frantic.

STUDENT: Right. Sometimes I do OK, but I feel so time-crunched and it doesn't help my work to get that stressed out about it.

COACH: I can understand that. Let's talk about what kind of strategies might help you get there. What kind of things are you doing now for a big project?

STUDENT: I check the syllabus. See when it's due.

COACH: OK. What do you do with that information?

STUDENT: Um, well, I'll put it in my planner that it's due, but my planner only shows a week at a time, so it's not like I keep checking it.

COACH: Gotcha. So it's in the planner, but because it's not in front of you for that week, it isn't really reminding you.

STUDENT: Yeah, I mean the professor will bring it up at times, but if I have other things going on, then I don't really work on it.

COACH: Right, and there are probably always other things that are going on. How about when you first see the assignment at the beginning of the semester? Do you think about it then?

STUDENT: Hmmm . . . I try not to be overwhelmed! I don't know, I see if it is a group project for sure, so that I know if I need to work with other people and that whole deal.

COACH: That changes things for sure. Let's say it is an individual project, like the one you have for biology this semester. I'm wondering if you think about how this single assignment might be divided into separate pieces that you can break apart and do in chunks.

STUDENT: Right, I see what you mean. Well, sometimes the professor will do that for you, divide it into smaller assignments so you stay on track that way.

COACH: OK, so what if the professor doesn't do that, what do you think about dividing it up into more manageable pieces? Or it can help if it feels more like a series of steps instead of just one big project.

STUDENT: Yeah, OK. I get that.

COACH: Go ahead and pull out your assignment for biology. Read through it and let's see if there is a logical way to divide it up.

From this point, the coach can become a scribe, writing down ideas about different components of the project as the student identifies them. The coach can cue the student to dig deeper if need be, for example, by having the student identify what might come before or after, or how chunks can be broken down even further (such as identifying resources or meeting with a subject librarian as an important step in doing research). Form 4.6 (Action Planning) is useful here.

A common need in this domain is *to develop tools to manage assignments and schedules*. This is particularly true for students just entering a postsecondary setting, who may already have some strategies for managing assignments, but less understanding of how they will manage their own schedule now that each day of the week is not a repeat of the previous day. Even students who are struggling to manage their time often have some strategies in place. It is up to the coach and student to figure out if the current strategies could be effective if they were better used, or if they should be abandoned for new ones. For example:

COACH: So you say you are having a hard time with your assignments and want to be able to know what you need to do. What are you doing now?

STUDENT: Well, I got this planner at the store, but I don't know, I guess I don't really use it. I mean, I open it and I think about using it sometimes, but when I sit down to do my work and look at it, it doesn't help.

COACH: OK, so you are looking at it when it comes time to do your homework, but it doesn't have what you need in it.

STUDENT: Yeah. I just have to look at my syllabus anyway, but then sometimes the assignments change.

COACH: Sure. Let's take a look at it. Do you have it with you?

STUDENT: Yeah, I keep it in my bag.

COACH: Great. OK, so it is just the date on each page and the lines with times. It doesn't look like you've written in here very much.

STUDENT: No. I mean, sometimes. Well, sometimes I'll use sticky notes and stick them on my books with what I need to read.

COACH: Oh, like Chapter 7 in this book, that kind of thing?

STUDENT: Yeah, then I don't have to look back at the syllabus, it's right there on the book.

COACH: OK, and how do you figure out what needs to go on the sticky notes?

STUDENT: I look at the syllabus, but sometimes I get it wrong because we get behind in class or the professor changes the reading. Or I've even started reading the same chapter twice because the sticky note was still there.

COACH: Ah. OK. So it sounds like you've got two strategies, but neither one is really working for you.

STUDENT: Yeah, I like the sticky notes, and I want to be able to just look at the planner to know what I need to do, but it doesn't work like that.

COACH: How about your planner—when do you usually add things to it?

STUDENT: Well, I guess that is part of the problem now that you mention it. I don't know. Sometimes during class? No, I'll put stuff in at the beginning of the semester, like big stuff, but then I try to add some stuff when I get home after class, but I guess I've forgotten by then, then I need to go look at the syllabus or my notes, and then I get overwhelmed. When are you supposed to write in those things?

In this example, the student has two strategies that are poorly formed—the planner and the sticky notes—but that can likely be retained if the student better understands how to use them. Questioning by the coach also revealed where the student was having difficulty, that is, in adding information to the planner, not in reviewing it. The student also described that the current planner felt hard to use and that when there were too many steps in the process, the strategy was abandoned. As the student and coach continued to talk, she mentioned that she also used the calendar on her phone a lot, particularly for errands, like going by the student union to get a bus pass. She would enter that errand into her calendar for a specific time and date. That way, a quick glance at the daily schedule of classes on her phone would also cue her to stop by the student union after her last class. Because her phone was a helpful tool in planning, the student decided to explore some options for apps that would sync with her daily calendar but allow her to enter specific to-do lists for classes.

While many students are relatively tech-savvy in that they are comfortable using smartphones, tablets, and laptops for schoolwork, these devices do not replace the work that the student and coach must do together to identify goals and matching strategies. For example, remember that the challenge for this student was knowing when to enter information about her assignments into her planner, and possibly knowing what that information needed to be so that she could complete the assignment later without needing to consult her notes or syllabus (if possible). The app itself does not address that problem, but using a device that is familiar and that the student is experiencing success with at similar activities (or errands) lays the foundation for the student to find success here as well.

Both Apple and Google have apps for to-do lists that have features such as timed alerts or geo-alerts that will send a notification when a person arrives at a location. They can also sync with calendars and can be organized into different lists or be tagged so that students can easily sort assignments by class or view all assignments and sort them by due date. Deciding which features are important and then developing training so that the student is able to enter information quickly and accurately often become a goal prerequisite to managing assignments and daily schedules.

Table 6.4 contains a few time-management apps that students have found useful. All have very similar features, but have differences in the interface that may make some more or less appealing to students. Together the coach and student should ensure that the app has features that address the student's needs (although these should be individualized, at a minimum, students need a place for due dates, assignment notes, sorting by class, etc.) and that the student is able to learn the interface easily. Depending on the level of the student's needs and familiarity with such applications, the student may be able to practice entering tasks during a coaching session, then have "homework" to enter all current assignments into the app before the next session. Students who require more support (particularly because of memory or learning needs) may spend the session developing a "cheat sheet" with the coach describing the steps to enter tasks, then initially practice in the presence of the coach so that accuracy of the assignments entered can be confirmed. Goals can progress through fading the support of the coach and then the "cheat sheet" as the process of task entering becomes well learned.

TABLE 6.4. Samples of Time-Management Applications

To-do lists	Sample features	Link
Reminders for iOS	• iOS only • Sync across devices • Geolocation • Organize under separate lists	*https://support.apple.com/en-us/HT205890*
Google Tasks	• Android or iOS • Sync across devices, including Google calendar • Link with email • Browser shortcuts	*https://chrome.google.com/webstore/detail/google-tasks-by-google/dmglolhoplikcoamfgjgammjbgchgjdd?hl=en*
"Better" Google Tasks	• Android or iOS • Add-on extension to Google tasks that improves user interface • Colors, different views by list and calendar	*https://chrome.google.com/webstore/detail/better-google-tasks/denjcdefjebbmlihdoojnebochnkgcin?hl=en-GB*
Finish	• iOS only • Designed to address procrastination • Short-, mid-, and long-term time frames • Set up alerts to work on projects (not just due dates)	*http://getfinish.com*
Any.Do	• Android only • Simple interface • Free • Sync across devices • Sync with calendar	*https://play.google.com/store/apps/details?id=com.anydo*
Pocket List	• iOS only • Sync across devices, including Apple Watch • Add icons for lists • Prioritize tasks • Stream shows all tasks by due date	*www.pocketlistsapp.com*
Remember the Milk	• Android or iOS • Shortcuts to add tasks • Multiple notification options (email, texts, alerts, Twitter, etc.) • Organize tasks into lists • Subtasks • Search function	*www.rememberthemilk.com*
Evernote	• Android or iOS • Integrate tasks with notes • Search function • Share • Tag tasks for quick sorting	*https://evernote.com*
Google Keep	• Android only • Integrate tasks with notes • Geolocation • Often preinstalled (no need to download)	*https://play.google.com/store/apps/details?id=com.google.android.keep*

(continued)

TABLE 6.4. *(continued)*

To-do lists	Sample features	Link
Listastic	• iOS • Sync with Apple Watch • Designed for sharing—good for group work • Drag-and-drop tasks between lists • Use gestures (swiping tasks)	*http://mcleanmobile.com/Listastic*
Trello	• Android or iOS • Create tasks as "cards" on "boards" • Drag and drop to organize • Add pictures to text • Visual cues to share, add due dates, subgoals, tags	*https://trello.com*

Other students prefer to stick with traditional paper-and-pen planners, but may still benefit from similar discussions with the coach to identify what features of assignments need to be entered in order for the planner to be useful. Unlike many of the apps we've mentioned, planners often have only blank spaces with each date, leaving it to the student to know what information needs to be entered so that tasks can be successfully completed. If a student enters in her planner "read Chapter 7—discussion in class" as it was specifically stated on a syllabus, it is unclear from looking at the planner what class the reading refers to (and therefore which book) and whether the note "discussion in class" refers to something that has already happened or that the student needs to prepare for and, if so, if this is a small group or classwide discussion. In this sense, students need careful strategy training to make planners effective tools.

In many cases, students can generate effective habits to do just that; in others, students have developed their own planners by identifying their needs, piloting self-made planners, making adjustments, and then using a local printing service to produce them. You may have noticed that this process follows the same strategize–act–adjust loop described as the GSAA cycle. A student who requires this level of specificity in a planner affords a coach with a good opportunity to explicitly teach this process on a large scale. However, whether a student chooses a mass-market planner or a digital app, the same GSAA process should guide him or her toward the current goal with an eye on how this process folds into future goal achievement.

Another useful time-management strategy is a prediction–performance contrast like the Plan–Do–Review shown in Form 6.1. This forms assists the student in becoming more accurate at monitoring the time commitment needed for various academic activities. Students list an activity, then predict how much time that activity will take. They then time themselves actually performing the activity and use the form to make a comparison. Students are often surprised to find that times vary widely depending on course subjects. Reading a chapter in a novel may take half an hour, but reading a chapter in a statistics or oceanography text may take much longer. The Plan–Do–Review process enables students to plan time more appropriately for their studies. Students also begin to understand that the goal of this activity is not to reduce the time spent studying, but to increase the accuracy of their predictions. Again, this process makes for a very achievable goal that sets the learner up for future success in planning as well.

Just as the student described in the previous section "Goal Setting in Self-Learning" needed to learn how to manage and write papers, students with executive function problems commonly struggle to manage long-term projects like presentations, papers, or book-length reading assignments. For such projects, students will not have enough opportunities to observe their performance as they did for discrete weekly assignments with the Plan–Do–Review. These long-term assignments necessitate starting the semester with a meeting between the coach and student to manage immediate needs, but as soon as possible, should move toward considering these semester-long projects. Just as writing a paper can be divided into discrete (if iterative) steps, students should be encouraged to divide large projects into smaller ones, along with subgoals and specific due dates. Because these types of assignments are so challenging to students with deficits in executive functioning, it can be easy for coaches to slip back into the didactic role of instructing students on how to manage a large project. Although some instruction may be necessary, coaches need to monitor their approach so that students clearly learn how to self-manage a large assignment, rather than only following the coaches' direction. Compare the following script with the one earlier in the chapter, and consider how this directive approach differs from a self-regulation coaching approach.

COACH: I see on your syllabus for biology that you have one lab project that you have to do as a group where you run an experiment. That sounds like it will be time-consuming.

STUDENT: Yeah, I haven't really done that before.

COACH: Sure. Is this your first biology course?

STUDENT: Yeah. I know one other person in that class though.

COACH: Oh good—you'll have to contact that person and set up a group. It says here that you need to meet with the lab instructor to get your research question approved. When do think you should schedule that?

STUDENT: Um, maybe by the end of the month?

COACH: OK, let's go ahead and put that meeting in your calendar, and then set up a reminder for you to schedule it with the lab instructor by email.

The coach here is *leading the student,* rather than guiding the student to find his or her own path. Below is a more elaborate example of how a coach may elicit the same action plan by *guiding the student* to consider past experiences in light of how he or she would like to see the current project progressing.

> COACH: So last week we talked a lot about your immediate needs to get your feet under you at the start of the semester. This week we are going to spend some time thinking more about your whole semester. How comfortable are you with your syllabi and what is expected of you in each of your classes?

> STUDENT: Oh, I've definitely looked through them a lot, but I'm not totally sure what I need to do. I mean, generally yes, but mostly I was getting textbooks and reading for this week. I did have one quiz.

> COACH: Some classes start quickly like that. [If quiz taking is related to a goal, the student and coach may want to explore this further.] Do you know of any big, long-term type projects that you'll have to do this semester?

> STUDENT: Um, yeah. I think so. (Hesitates.)

> COACH: If you're unsure, feel free to check your syllabi. We can look at them together if you'd like.

> STUDENT: Okay great, yeah, I was thinking I had something for biology. Huh. It looks like a lab project of some kind.

> COACH: Yeah, I see that. It looks like it is worth 20% of your grade too, so that's a nice place you could earn points. How do you do with managing big projects like this? Have you had success in the past?

> STUDENT: Yeah, well, I've done okay. Well, honestly, I get pretty stressed out about them, but I've done okay. This one is completely new though, so it does worry me.

> COACH: Right; I can see that. Well, the other thing to remember about these types of projects is that the course should be teaching you how to do it at the same time that you are doing it. Does that make sense? Like, right now you don't know how to do it because you haven't taken biology before, but it looks like you have a lab report that you'll do during lab next week, so maybe you'll feel better once you've got some practicing under your belt.

> STUDENT: True. Yeah, I get that.

> COACH: So what are your thoughts about how to manage a big project? What kinds of things have you done in the past?

> STUDENT: You mean, like in other classes?

COACH: Yeah, tell me about that.

STUDENT: I definitely check the syllabus. It's super helpful when the professor goes over it in class, and sometimes gives you a handout that tells you what to do and how it will be scored. Those are the ones I felt best about.

COACH: Sure, it's nice to have it all spelled out for you. Then you can use it almost like a checklist: have I done this, have I done that?

STUDENT: Yeah, those are the best.

COACH: So there's a good chance that you will talk more about this project and even get a handout about it. But let's say that you don't. Is there enough here in your syllabus that you could make a handout like that?

STUDENT: Like, a list of what I need to do?

COACH: Yeah, exactly. What do you think?

STUDENT: Um, maybe. Well, some things yeah. Like I see there's a deadline to pick a topic and get it approved, so I could put that there.

COACH: Great. Good start. Let's see what else we can go ahead and spell out. Do you want to write these down, or would you like me to take some notes for you?

This approach is clearly more labor intensive and lengthier for both coach and student, but the trade-off is that students lead the process so that they learn how to manage their own learning.

MANAGING INEFFECTIVE STRATEGIES

Students who have ABIs often have maladaptive routines in place that may have worked well enough before an injury but that have now become ineffective after cognitive changes. For other students with executive function problems, strategies may also have been largely unnecessary because of the support structure provided in secondary educational settings. Now faced with the demands of college, students often rely on poorly formed notions of strategic learning. Two ineffective strategies from the self-learning and self-management domains that we encountered repeatedly were use of repetition to learn material ("I just do it again and again") and procrastinating on assignments as a time-management approach ("I'll get to that later, when the due date is closer," or "It'll get done one way or the other"). Although neither of these strategies is effective, to a young adult, they likely met the threshold of being just effective enough to hold onto them. For example, a good learner might go back and review notes to study and perhaps recite them aloud to encode the information, and then do fairly well on a quiz (e.g., well enough that the student is satisfied with his or her performance and feels that it is not neces-sary to adapt the strategy). However, what this student does not realize is that it is unlikely that the repetition alone led to an adequate performance.

Although you may not think of procrastination as a strategy, students have so many demands on their time that procrastination often amounts to developing a to-do list based on priority or the task that is due next (colloquially, whichever task is screaming the loudest). It is a passive form of time management: "I'll do that when the time comes, because right now I am thinking about this other thing that I have to do right away." The schedule is set so that tasks are done right before they are due and not before. Our students at times acknowledged that this strategy is difficult to overcome for two reasons: (1) it requires effortful planning and, even more important, (2) it may have been effective in the past. Students could have been staying up all night to complete assignments or waiting until the last minute and still earned grades that were acceptable enough that there was no need to self-adjust their self-regulation loop. In effect, actual performance was close enough to their goal performance that they were likely to approach the next assignment the same way.

The procrastination strategy clearly will not work for individuals with execu-tive function problems in postsecondary educational settings for a number of rea-sons. Just as students with these problems reported needing more time to review material, they also need more time to finish most tasks. In addition, students (in general) are often poor judges of how much time is needed before a due date to complete an assignment and frequently do not allocate enough. In the general population, this is known as the planning fallacy (Kahneman & Tversky, 1979), in which people are overly optimistic about the conditions that surround the task at hand. In individuals with executive function problems, this is compounded by the fact that they may still be learning how their cognition works in a college set-ting, so that estimates of the time needed to complete tasks are very inaccurate. Second, students with brain injuries often struggle with fatigue and must employ good sleep habits to maximize cognition. Staying up late working on assignments or cramming, therefore, doubly works against them, both by giving them less time than they need to complete a quality product and also by robbing them of their best cognitive efforts on subsequent days.

However, there is a huge amount of inertia behind use of strategies that have been used in the past. Students want to continue using the strategies that they are comfortable with because implementing new ones can feel like adding more work to the work that they are already trying to accomplish. Goals may, therefore, need to address the extinction or expansion of current strategies rather than suggest-ing a replacement and expecting it to take the place of an ingrained routine. For example, if the student is using repetition with flashcards, this can be expanded through the student self-quizzing (retrieval practice), sorting cards by familiarity (monitoring of learning), or using the vocabulary word in a sentence (elaborative encoding). Therefore, the existing strategy of repetition is not only linked to more effective memorization techniques, enhancing the effectiveness of learning, but it also increases the likelihood of the student actually enacting the strategies. Coaches can also take the opportunity to explain the stages of memorization (i.e., encoding, storage, retrieval) and how these added techniques address these stages and result in more effective learning. With appropriate support, students may be able to identify these strategies independently as the coach describes the steps needed for effective recall of learned material.

This educational component can be important for students with executive function problems. In order for these students to "learn how they learn," coaches need to provide information on cognitive processes (see Table 1.1) and how they are affected by executive function problems (see Table 1.2). Here, the old saying "Knowledge is power" can be applied. The more students understand how learning and planning occur, the more they can exert some control over them by developing strategies that target their needs.

TAKING ACTION: TRACKING STRATEGIES AND PERFORMANCE IN SELF-LEARNING AND SELF-MANAGEMENT

Goal setting and even strategizing are often quite familiar to students, but having students use their strategies and make adjustments to strategies (Act and Adjust, in Goal–Strategize–Act–Adjust) are critical pieces of intervention that are equally important. Students may know that they will be expected to work on their goals between intervention sessions but may be surprised that coaches want them to track this work. Tracking the use of strategies is important for a few reasons. First, students are more likely to actually use their strategies if they know they need to be keeping track of them and will be showing the tracking record to the coach at the next meeting. Second, students will have a better idea as to what worked about a strategy and what did not if they have charted their strategy use across the intervening time period. Third, this tracking then leads to more effective adjustment of strategies so that goals can be met. Fourth, tracking specifically teaches students to self-monitor so that students become used to checking whether they are using the strategies in their toolkits and if those strategies are meeting their needs.

Form 4.4, Tracking Strategy Action, helps students to track strategy use between each session. Tracking starts on a Monday of a typical school week, but can be adjusted to start with each coaching session if need be. Each day, the student rates whether or not a strategy was necessary and the degree to which it was used. The student can also use the final column to note any barriers to or successes with strategy use. Alternatively, the student could use a system of +/−, with each rating to indicate on which particular days the strategies went smoothly versus other days for which the strategies were more challenging. Although the coach and student will explore this tracking and strategy use in more detail during weekly sessions, this form provides a snapshot of how the student used the strategies during the week. For example, if a strategy has mostly zeros, indicating that it was not necessary, then it may be that this strategy is not meeting the student's needs or that it is not targeting the performance goal directly enough.

Mobile applications are also available to track strategy use throughout the week. These apps are open ended, allowing students to enter their personal strategies, then track them using number systems or emoticons. Helpfully, many of these apps have reminder alerts so that students may complete their tracking at multiple times during the day. These apps tend to cluster under the title of "Habit Trackers." Examples include:

- Habit List (*http://habitlist.com*)
- Productive (*http://productiveapp.io*)
- HabitBull (*www.habitbull.com*)
- Strides (*www.stridesapp.com*)
- Momentum (*http://momentum.cc*)
- Streaks (*http://streaksapp.com*)
- Daily Goals (*http://cascodelabs.com/#dailygoals*)
- Goals on Track (*www.goalsontrack.com*)

Of course, the challenge is that the more open ended the app, the more complex it will be to learn. Coaches should proceed with care in recommending these apps, reserving them only for students who prefer using this technology and are already successfully using it for other tasks, such as their daily calendar. Apps from this list that provide a more basic interface include *Productive* and *Streaks*. *Streaks* allows only six items to be entered, so that the user can focus on achieving a manageable set of goals. More complex interfaces, such as *Goals on Track,* link habit tracking to goals. Preferably, if the coach has an Android and iOS device available, it can be loaded with such apps for the student to explore during the session. If this is not possible, coaches should still educate themselves about these options to be able to recommend a limited set from which the student can select (i.e., a quick Google search shows thousands of such apps—the student will appreciate not needing to select from them all)

Just as some students may choose to monitor their class performance by creating a spreadsheet of the grading system from the syllabus, other students may prefer to use a spreadsheet to track strategy use. Students can list strategies, provide ratings or frequency counts, and write detailed notes if they so choose. More experienced users can use graphs to show consistency of usage over time. With the advent of Google Sheets, these strategies could also be shared with coaches, allowing for even greater transparency between sessions.

Because strategy tracking is secondary to strategy use, it is important that whatever tracking system is selected feels very easy and manageable to use and places minimal demands on students' already limited time. Ideally, students will find tracking rewarding. Seeing the accumulation of the student's efforts summarized on the tracking sheet, app, or spreadsheet can provide a pleasant visual reminder of the progress being made toward goals.

ADJUSTMENT: STRATEGY USEFULNESS AND NEXT STEPS

During coaching sessions, adjustments are linked explicitly to monitoring, which has been facilitated by tracking strategy use between sessions. As students progress, they may be able to adjust strategies independently between sessions, particularly by making small modifications to fit the context of application. At least initially, though, coaches should expect discussions around this component to be a large part of each session. Most adjustments will address the level of the strategy, but can also modify the plan (strategy implementation) or goal itself. Each of these will be described below.

Coaches and students will find Form 4.4, Tracking Strategy Action, Form 4.5, Strategy Usefulness and Next Steps, and Form 4.7, Student Summary of Strategies helpful in considering successes, barriers, and next step adjustments. Form 4.4 can be used by the coach to determine the extent to which the student is using (and reporting on the use of) strategies. For students who are ready to evaluate the usefulness of a strategy with a fair amount of ease, Form 4.5 will be helpful. However, Form 4.7 serves to consider the expenditure-versus-gain tradeoff for students who may be ambivalent about a new strategy. When a new strategy is initiated, it can be expected that it will be more effortful to complete, but over time, those ratings should decrease. If not, the coach will want to query the student about implementation and the conditions in which the strategy is being used. One architecture student struggled to use a smartpen (*www.livescribe.com/en-us/smartpen/echo/*) to record his notes during class. As explained earlier, this pen records audio that syncs with the position of the pen on the page, so that touching a particular spot on the pen will replay the audio that occurred as the student recorded those notes. The student still felt pressured to keep up with professor, even though the pen would allow him to record notes at his own pace, then return to them after class to fill in missing details. It is unsurprising that the breakthrough came when he slightly adjusted his strategy so that rather than recording the professor's lecture verbatim in his notes, he began interspersing his notes with drawings. Since the pen could recall the audio just as easily from these drawings as from written words, the strategy adjustment allowed him time to catch up with the lecture and the drawings linked what he was hearing to visual cues. Although his daily tracking form (Form 4.4) showed little change, this slight adjustment to his strategy implementation led to a reduction in effort and an increase in "how helpful" the strategy was (Form 4.7). Movement on those two measures led to a highly valued strategy that was carried over to the other classes and future semesters (Form 4.8).

Another example may be helpful here. One student found it effortful to schedule group meetings with other students to review ahead of exams. It was a lot of time and work, and she had to be flexible, something with which she struggled. The coach used Form 4.7 to find out how she viewed this activity; it turned out that she evaluated it as a lot of work and effort, but very important given the gaps in her knowledge base that peers could help to fill in. An effortful strategy may be retained if the student recognizes that it is improving performance significantly. Furthermore, this form allows students and coaches to see the pattern of self-appraisal reveals that nearly all new strategies are effortful at first, but with time, and as the strategy becomes more routine, they become less effortful.

Form 4.5 provides a structured framework for coaches and students to discuss whether and how to make adjustments to strategies, plans, or goals. A student may decide to modify a reading strategy so that instead of highlighting a text, she is using a pen to jot notes in the margin. If she chose to adjust the plan, she may instead need more direction about how and when to use the strategy, using highlighting for all of her reading assignments rather than only English literature, or to have her highlighters with her in her backpack, so that if she chooses to do her reading at the library, she has the tools she needs.

In most cases, it is best to reserve altering the goal until the strategy or plan has been thoroughly explored. However, in some cases, the student may be becoming more realistic about his or her abilities or shifting priorities. For those students, adjusting a goal can be appropriate and can indicate some progress toward improved monitoring and updating of metacognitive beliefs. As an example, a student had set a goal of earning all As in his courses. By the middle of the semester, he realized that doing so was likely unattainable, or that at the least, that it was taking a toll on his well-being. He was spending all of his time studying, and had developed a habit of checking and rechecking his work, so that he might look at the same assignment more than a dozen times to ensure that it was correct. He was also avoiding his roommates and their offers to participate in social events. He decided to reduce his goal to allow for some Bs and instead added a social-participation goal (see Chapter 7 for more discussion of these goals). At the end of the semester, he had both As and Bs and had joined an intramural softball team. By modifying his self-learning goal, he had allowed himself to simultaneously meet an important self-advocacy goal as well.

Chapter 7 covers self-advocacy in more depth, but we should continue to keep in mind how the three domains of self-learning, self-management, and self-advocacy overlap and can be used to support one another. Just as effective self-management allows a student to plan appropriate time for studying, students need to be able to advocate for their academic and social needs. The GSAA process laid out here remains the same, though—students are best served by learning how to monitor and manage their own learning.

ADDITIONAL RESOURCES

- A sample of online study skill resources are available through college websites and independent websites. Here is a sampling:
  - *www.dartmouth.edu/~acskills/handouts.html*
  - *https://dus.psu.edu/academicsuccess/studyskills.html*
  - *http://academictips.org*
- For learning how to instruct students in specific strategies who have moderate to severe memory and attention deficits and need more intensive cognitive rehabilitation therapy, see *Optimizing Cognitive Rehabilitation* by Sohlberg and Turkstra (2011) and *Cognitive Rehabilitation Manual: Translating Evidence-Based Recommendations into Practice* by Haskins and colleagues (2012).
- For students with more severe cognitive and behavioral impairments, see the book *Collaborative Brain Injury Intervention* by Ylvisaker and Feeney (1998) and a systematic review by Ylvisaker and colleagues (2007).
- For systematic reviews and best practice for using memory strategies, see Velikonja and colleagues (2014) and O'Neil-Pirozzi and colleagues (2016).
- For a review of cognitive rehabilitation therapy for military service and veterans, see *Cognitive Rehabilitation Therapy for Traumatic Brain Injury* (Institute of Medicine, 2011).

Plan–Do–Review

PLAN			DO		REVIEW
Due date/priority	Task description	Time expected	Check	Actual time	Comments/observations

CHAPTER 7

Coaching Self-Advocacy

Self-advocacy consists of a set of knowledge and skills that includes understanding your strengths and needs, identifying your personal goals, knowing your legal rights and responsibilities, and having the ability to communicate this knowledge to others (*http://www.greatschools.org/gk/articles/self-advocacy-teenager-with-ld*). Self-advocacy skills are critically important for college students with executive function problems, regardless of whether or not the disability is newly acquired. In Chapter 5, readers learned how coaches can assist students in understanding and interpreting their cognitive and executive function strengths and weaknesses, and also learned how to coach students in how to identify and create their own academic goals. In Chapter 6, readers learned how to coach students to create measurable goals; create plans and identify strategies; put strategies into action and track the results; assess the results; and modify goals, strategies, and plans if needed, as these skills are related to managing time, being organized, and studying and learning.

Self-advocacy is based on a sound and accurate perception of oneself. As students are coached in college, they begin to experience and learn about their abilities and disabilities; these experiences help them become better advocates because they come to understand themselves more deeply and more broadly. Indeed, "awareness" improves by having varied experiences (Tate et al., 2014). The coach's job is now to align students' knowledge of themselves with self-advocacy skills that suit their personality and communication style. The focus of this chapter, therefore, is on coaching students so that they can advocate not only for educational services and accommodations, but also for other needs with friends and family. The objectives of this chapter are to:

- Explain how self-advocacy is related to other personal factors that contribute to students' reluctance and resistance to seeking help.
- Describe self-advocacy within the context of accommodations and the rights of college students with executive function problems.
- Describe coaching using the GSAA approach to self-advocacy with supportive teams of individuals and with friends and peers.

WHAT COACHES NEED TO KNOW ABOUT SELF-ADVOCACY IN COLLEGE STUDENTS

It cannot be emphasized enough that self-advocacy skills are a necessity for all college students with disabilities. The value of self-advocacy is supported not only by research evidence, but is also confirmed by my own practice-based experiences. Students who self-advocate are more likely to be successful in college. Self-advocacy is a critical skill that predicts grade point average among students with disabilities over many other variables (Janiga & Costenbader, 2002; Lombardi et al., 2011). Furthermore, the transition from high school to college is easier for those who self-advocate (e.g., Beauchamp & Kiewra, 2004).

But self-advocacy is also related to personal development. Walker (2010) investigated relationships between self-advocacy, career maturity, and career decision making in college students with and without disabilities. She found that students *without disabilities were higher in career maturity and self-advocacy* than were students with disabilities; and that for the *students with disabilities, those with high self-advocacy were higher in career maturity than those with lower self-advocacy.*

In my work with this group of students, I have found that they are reluctant to self-advocate and are unsure of how to go about it. The reasons for this are described shortly, and may be similar to the reasons that college students with other kinds of disabilities do not self-advocate. Yet having problems with executive function means that these students may not be able to plan, strategize, and implement a plan without the support and instruction of a coach. Knowing about the following personal barriers to self-advocacy helps coaches understand and anticipate why students appear reluctant.

1. College students with disabilities, including those with executive function problems, may not have *self-advocacy skills simply because they were not needed (and therefore not developed) in the past*. Students who are transitioning from high school to college likely had others advocating for them. The support they received did not rely on their own self-advocacy, but on the advocacy of their parents and teachers. Simply put, self-advocacy skills were not learned.

Students with a newly acquired disability (e.g., TBI, stroke, multiple sclerosis) typically received medical-based rehabilitation with a good deal of support and encouragement from healthcare professionals. The goals of rehabilitation specialists are to repair, heal, and treat the individual so that she or he can become as successful as possible. Family and friends' involvement in rehabilitation is encouraged because we know that individuals with a support system have better outcomes than those without one. This medical model works well when students are ill, but falls short when dealing with a chronic condition in college. College educators' goals are to promote independence, self-expression, and "finding your own way." Support is given to students with disabilities *if they seek it, if they request it.* When these students and their parents and medical professionals are not aware of the expectations that the college culture places on students, misunderstandings and lack of follow-through can result in students not receiving the supports they are entitled to by law.

2. *Self-advocacy is related to other personal factors as well.* In particular, help-seeking behaviors of adolescent students with disabilities has been *linked to self-perception, having goals, coping strategies, and the cost/benefits of seeking help.* In a 1997 study of adolescents' reports of asking for help with math, Ryan and Pintrich found that students with low self-perception of their cognitive and social skills were less likely to ask for help, that is, more likely be avoidant. In a more recent study, Hartman-Hall and Haaga (2002) investigated relationships between self-perception of disability, types of goals, professors' responses (negative, positive), and the willingness of students with learning disabilities to seek help. College students with learning disabilities reported a willingness to seek help *when professors' responses were positive* and an unwillingness to seek help (i.e., avoid doing so) when professors' responses were negative. Furthermore, students who viewed their *disability as changeable and without stigma (i.e., those with high self-esteem) were more likely to report a willingness to ask for help* than students who perceived their disability as unchangeable, "global," and negative (i.e., low self-esteem) (p. 263). Finally, the kinds of goals had some influence on whether these students asked for help; specific and measurable goals (e.g., improved grades) were associated with help seeking, whereas general goals (e.g., improved learning) were associated with avoidance behavior.

Students who have a negative self-perception, or perceive their disability as a stigma, may feel threatened when their self-advocacy results in a negative response. In other words, a stigma can be confirmed in the mind of the student who feels threatened when getting a negative response (or a perceived negative response) from the professor. On the other hand, when students with positive self-perceptions receive a negative response, they are more likely to attribute that response to circumstances that have nothing to do with them. Consider the following example. A student who has stigmatized her disability approaches the professor after class to discuss the logistics for getting extended time on the upcoming exam. The professor is packing up class materials and says to the student, "Can we talk about this after the next class? I don't have time right now. I have to get to a meeting." The stigmatized student may think, "See, I knew this would be a hassle. I'm so embarrassed. I knew I couldn't figure out how to do this. He really doesn't want to help me." This exact same scenario involving a student who has a strong self-perception could be interpreted differently, as "Oh, this professor was really busy today. I'll approach him after the next class, like he asked me to do." In the latter scenario, the student has taken the professor's response at face value and has not personalized it, as the first student had done.

3. *Students may be reluctant to ask for help because it conflicts with striving to be independent.* After all, during their time in college students become less dependent on their family and seek to align more closely with peers. Developmentally, this is a critically significant phase that includes neurobiological changes (e.g., completion of the frontal lobe and its connections), social changes (e.g., exploring various social groups to find where one belongs), and intellectual changes (e.g., exploring interests, identifying job and career paths).

Yet, for students with executive function problems, this developmental period frequently has the additional challenges of not quite having the skills necessary to become "independent," which is what these students—and their peers—aspire to. They have the same desire to become independent as do other students with or without disabilities. Students who have received accommodations before entering college may view this time as an opportunity to get off "the disability track." They may have a wait-and-see attitude: "I'll get help if I need it." Students with a newly acquired executive function problem, however, have little previous experience with asking for help, nor do they know what and/or if they are going need help, given their lack of experience living with their new disabilities and preserved abilities. To complicate this further, these students are being forced back into more dependent relationships with their family because of their injury or illness, which is the very opposite of the trajectory toward independence. These factors, coupled with misperceptions about the roles and responsibilities of disability services, keep nearly 50% of these students from getting the coaching support and services that are available and that they are entitled to receive (Kennedy et al., 2008).

4. *Students with disabilities may not register with disability services because of misperceptions about who uses these services and what services are offered.* Consider these comments from students who are discussing disability services:

> "Isn't that like being in special education? I don't need special ed."

> "I thought those services were only for people who are hearing impaired, blind, or use a wheelchair. You know, like if you need an interpreter."

> "I don't need lots of help, just a little. That's [disability services] for students who need a lot more help than I do."

"I didn't qualify for special ed in high school, so I didn't think I'd qualify for those services now that I'm in college."

"I didn't even know there was this kind of help on campus."

"I don't even know what disability services can do for someone like me."

Table 7.1 lists the basic roles and responsibilities of college students, disability specialists, and instructors. It is vitally important that students and parents know and understand what each individual's role is in ascertaining reasonable

TABLE 7.1. Basic Roles and Responsibilities of Students, Disability Service Providers, and Instructors

Students	Disability services	Instructors
Provide medical and/or psychological documentation to disability services.	Educate students about what disability services does, including students' roles and responsibilities.	Refer students to disability services; participate in the process to determine accommodations.
Participate in the process of determining and implementing accommodations.	Determine if a condition is a disability based on professional reports.	Make sure that accommodations are being implemented as planned.
Inform and discuss with disability services if their disability changes.	Maintain medical/ psychological documentation in a confidential manner.	Use inclusive language in the course syllabus and during class to encourage students with disabilities to seek help when needed.
Inform and discuss with disability services when accommodations are not being implemented.	Identify and authorize accommodations to provide "access" but not necessarily academic "success."	Identify essential course components for accommodations to be determined.
Inform and discuss with disability services accommodations that are not working and that need to be modified.	Create a plan that includes accommodations and additional campus services.	Request assistance from disability services when questions or concerns occur.
Stay in contact with disability services periodically throughout the semester and academic year.	Assist with the implementation of reasonable accommodations; modify accommodations when needed.	Validate students' participation in class by calling on them when they offer comments or have questions.
Notify disability services when they are struggling in a course to create a plan.	Advocate for students with instructors and others, with students' permission.	When arranging group work or projects outside of class, ensure that the students' accommodations are being adhered to by checking in with students.

accommodations. It is worth noting that the student him- or herself is the one responsible for initiating contact with the disability services office; parents, rehabilitation specialists, and transition specialists can be involved in the process, but without the student's consent, the services will not be provided. That is, students themselves must take the initiative in the process of contacting and registering with these services. In this sense, *registering with disability services is an initial first step at becoming a self-advocate.*

STUDENT RIGHTS, RESPONSIBILITIES, AND SELF-ADVOCACY SKILLS

Most of us are aware of, if not familiar with, the Rehabilitation Act of 1973, Section 504, a federal law enacted to protect students with disabilities against discrimination, and to provide them equal access to education, including college. This law mandated that colleges provide reasonable accommodations in order for them to access the same education and services that students without disabilities have. The intention of this law is to level the playing field by providing equal access to education. In 1990, the Americans with Disabilities Act (ADA) reinforced the mandate for accommodations by extending it to public places. Accommodations are identified and authorized by trained staff at student disability services offices on college campuses. In 2008, revisions to the ADA broadened the definitions of disability to include mental or physical disabilities that limit individuals' participation in major life activities, and were embodied in the Americans with Disabilities Act Amendment Act (ADAAA). At the same time the U.S. Equal Employment Opportunity Commission (EEOC) was required to revise job and educational regulations to reflect the ADAAA; these regulations were approved in 2011 (*www.eeoc.gov/laws/ regulations/adaaa_fact_sheet.cfm*).

Cory (2011) summarized two key aspects of these laws that are essential for coaches, students, and college educators to understand. The first is *protection from discrimination while upholding "essential elements"* of a college program, major, or course. For example, traditional lecture hall classrooms with fluorescent lights may result in inattention, headaches, and fatigue for a student with PCS. Rather than dimming the lights for all students (which, in some cases, is reasonable and acceptable), a student may wear darkened sunglasses in class as an accommodation identified by a disability specialist. Let's say, though, that the instructor tells the student that she has a policy that no sunglasses can be worn in her classroom. This would be an example of unintentional discrimination that is not essential to learning and participating in the course. In other words, wearing sunglasses in class actually provides equal access to classroom learning for this student, without interfering with the essential learning. This problem could be avoided if the student shared his or her need for accommodations with the instructor, as it is the student's responsibility to do so.

However, there are some kinds of knowledge and skills that all students must have, called "essential elements" of a program, major, or course, for which no accommodations can be made. For example, students in speech–language graduate programs must meet acceptable speaking standards themselves, since their job as speech–language pathologists will involve assessing, modeling, and treating individuals with speech impairments. Because proficiency in language and speech is an essential element of these training programs, students with language or speech impairments may not be acceptable candidates for graduate school. Another example is learning course material for tests. Since the ability to recall information is an essential element of many college courses, students with working memory impairments who cannot retain material for an exam, even with reasonable accommodations (e.g., extended time, alternative test format), may not be able to complete the course.

A second key aspect to understand, according to Cory (2011), is that *accommodations must be reasonable*. Accommodations are modifications or adjustments to a course, program, service, job, facility, or activity that enables an otherwise qualified student with a disability to have an equal opportunity to participate. But the meaning of "reasonable" for college students "varies from class to class and person to person. What is reasonable for one student in a course may or may not be reasonable for another student in that same course, or for a student with the same disability in a different class. This is why accommodations are determined through a dialogue with students, DS staff, and instructors on a case-by-case basis" (Cory, 2011, p. 29).

Figure 7.1 illustrates the percentage of postsecondary institutions that provide various kinds of accommodations. These data (Raue & Lewis, 2011) were taken from 3,680 institutions that reported enrolling students with disabilities across the United States. The majority of institutions reported that they offer additional exam time (93%), note takers, study skill instruction, notes/assignments from instructors, alternative exam formats, adaptive equipment/technology, digitally recorded texts, readers, physical changes to classrooms, and tutors. Disability specialists determine accommodations based on reports and recommendations from neuropsychologists and other professionals. It is important to note that there is variability in the kinds of reports that are required, however, most institutions require reports of tests done by a licensed psychologist, although some will accept reports from speech–language pathologists, occupational therapists, and vocational psychologists as long as this kind of testing is within a discipline's scope of practice statewide and nationally.

The following short list of accommodations is typical of the kinds of modifications offered to college students with executive function problems. Note that accommodations that could be provided for other disabilities that students may

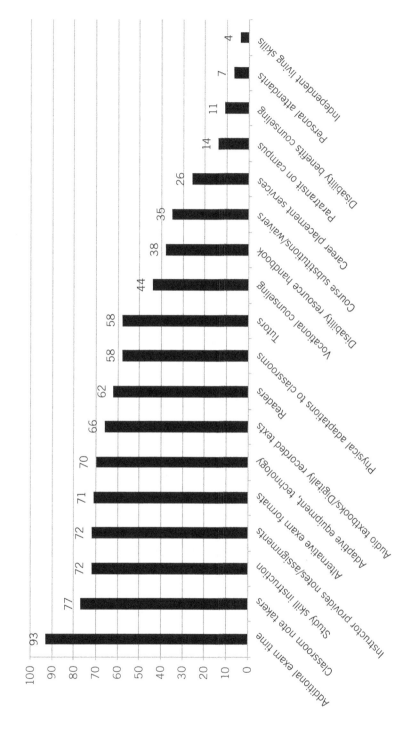

FIGURE 7.1. The percentage of postsecondary institutions that provide these specific accommodations to college students (Raue & Lewis, 2011).

197

have in addition to deficits with executive function, such as slow processing, memory impairment, reading impairment, and visual disability, are not listed.

- Extended time on exams
- Private, quiet space to take exams
- Extended time on assignments
- Note takers
- Instructor provides notes/assignments prior to class
- Using assistive technology

Regardless of which accommodations are authorized, they need to be frequently reviewed and modified so they reflect the kinds of changes students experience over the course of their time in college (Scott, 2002). But before any modifications can be arranged, students, disability specialists, program directors, and instructors need to have conversations about the following issues:

- What is reasonable given the essential elements of a program and the courses required.
- Whether or not accommodations are being implemented and, if so, are the accommodations providing equal access?

This iterative process requires that students meet and talk with their disability specialist on a regular basis, and not only at the beginning of the academic year, as so many students do. The second half of this chapter explains how students can be coached to work with disability specialists and instructors and peers.

COACHING SELF-ADVOCACY USING THE GSAA APPROACH

Coaching students with executive function problems to self-advocate must take into account students' self-perceptions, how they manage, interpret, and respond to negative responses from others, and the risks involved in doing so. They need to self-advocate not only with educators (e.g., disability service specialists, teaching assistants, and instructors), but also with their peers, friends, and family. In the next section, we start by describing how students can create a team of supporters as a self-advocacy activity. This discussion is followed by a description of the GSAA approach that coaches students to advocate for themselves in a manner that reflects their strengthening self-perception, self-efficacy, and their own personal communication style.

A Team Approach That Fosters Self-Advocacy

My work with college students has shown that for students with executive function problems having a supportive team has been vital to their success. In fact, students who create a supportive team are performing an act of self-advocacy. It is an explicit acknowledgment by the student that support beyond that given by a coach is needed. For this reason, having students create a team should be a coaching priority. There are two primary principles that coaches should keep in mind as students select and work with members of their team.

> PRINCIPLE 1. *Students identify the individual members of their team and acknowledge their need for support.*

Coaches can educate students about the roles and responsibilities of various professionals on campus and make recommendations, but ultimately, students make their own choices. This reinforces students' autonomy in deciding whom they want on their team. Table 7.2 lists potential team members who can be found on campus and other individuals who are a part of students' personal life off campus.

How can a coach start the conversation about teams with these students? The following is an example of a student who had difficulty with attention, affecting her ability to stay organized.

> COACH: There are quite a few individuals here on campus whom you rely on for various things, right? So, here is a list just to get you thinking about who you might want on your team. (*Shows the student the list in Table 7.2.*)
>
> STUDENT: OK, but what's the purpose of having a team again?
>
> COACH: Well, these are individuals who have a specific role or job to do in supporting you in college. Team members count on each other to be able to do their job. For example, you are counting on Jim, your disability specialist, to ensure that you get the accommodations the two of you had discussed.

TABLE 7.2. A List of Potential Team Members for Students to Consider

College-affiliated individuals	Individuals not affiliated with college
Coach	Family (parents, siblings)
Disability service provider	Friends, peers
Instructor	Vocational rehabilitation counselor
Advisor	Healthcare provider (e.g., occupational therapist, speech–language pathologist)
Mental health counselor	
Tutor	Mental health counselor
	Personal trainer

Here's a list of the kinds of people you might want on your team (*referring to Table 7.2 again*). You can use this form [Form 7.1] to list the individual, his or her relationship to you, and what she or he will do for you. You can put the individual's contact information here as well, just to keep it all organized and in one place.

STUDENT: So I can have other people on the team too, like my vocational counselor?

COACH: Of course.

STUDENT: Let's add my parents to the team and my best friend, Cheryl. I think that's it.

COACH: OK, let's see if there are others who are here on campus that you would like on the team (*Points to the list*). What do you think?

STUDENT: Definitely Jim from disability services. What about my Spanish instructor, who is even willing to meet me for coffee so I can practice my conversational skills?

Students typically invite family or close friends to be on their team, but many need suggestions from coaches to include other professionals who are in a good position to offer specific kinds of support, such as vocational counselors and disability specialists suggested by the coach in the above example.

Coaches should be aware that there is wide variation in the composition of teams. For some students, having family and friends join a team of mostly campus professionals is a priority. Other students are less connected to their family and may want only campus staff and faculty on their team. Unfortunately, some students do not want to explicitly identify a group of individuals as "a team," even though they are getting support and services from the group. While students' reasons vary, this decision may reflect a strong need for independence; however, for these students to be successful, they will need compensatory memory and organizational skills to keep track of what they need, when they need it, and from whom.

PRINCIPLE 2. *Teamwork allows students to see advocacy in action while they practice self-advocacy skills with supportive individuals in a safe environment where (for the most part) positive responses are anticipated.*

The formation of a team also allows coaches to model self-advocacy. Consider the conversation below.

COACH: I see you've listed your disability service specialist as a team member. It will be really helpful to have her on your team. You'll be able to keep her informed about how well the accommodations are working.

STUDENT: Oh, my accommodations can change? I thought you get them at the beginning of the year and that's it.

COACH: Actually, if for any reason the accommodations are not being implemented or if they are simply not working, you can talk to her. She knows better than I do how they can be changed and what is reasonable. With her on the team, all of this becomes much easier since she really knows you and what you are trying to do.

The amount and kind of coaching that students need to set up a team vary depending on students' executive function abilities. In the section that follows, we start off by describing how coaches can support students when creating a team by using the GSAA approach. We then turn to considerations to bear in mind when coaching students' self-advocacy with friends and peers.

Applying GSAA to Coaching Self-Advocacy

Let's use the GSAA approach to self-advocacy by describing how to coach students in team building, wherein the focus is on *communicating with disability service specialists, instructors, and other college staff.* In a complex activity such as this, the *self-regulation goal* is to have the student create and work with a team of individuals, whereas the *performance goal* is to have the student be able to explain what they need. The Action-Planning Form (Form 4.6) is well suited for this kind of activity because it provides a structure in which the steps can be written out by students with coaching support as needed. Thus, the *strategy* used here *is* the formulation and implementation of these self-identified steps. Having students predict how challenging each step will be and reflecting back on whether their prediction was correct forces them to activate the self-regulation feedback loop, thereby gaining a deeper understanding of their performance for future reference. Figure 7.2 illustrates this process for a student who is creating a support team.

With deadlines assigned to each step, the student had little difficulty following through (*act*). Although nothing needed *adjustment* to meet this goal, he learned several additional skills that would be useful in other situations, such as:

- How to describe what he needed and identify other situations in which explaining his needs would be useful (e.g., approaching instructors about their accommodation).
- How to use an online scheduling system.
- Anticipating how hard each step would be and how much time each step would take to complete.

Goal: *To invite individuals from various areas of my life to be members of my college team.*

Steps in my plan	Done (✓)	E = easy; R = routine; H = hard	
		Will be . . .	Was
1. *Identify individuals and describe their roles.* [Form 7.1] Due date: *1 week*	✓	*E*	*E*
2. *Get contact information for each individual.* [Form 7.1] Due date: 1 week	✓	*R*	*R*
3. *Write out why I am forming a team and what I would like them to do. Write this in an email to each individual.* Due date: 2 weeks	✓	*E*	*H*
4. *Create a finalized list of team members based on their response.* Due date: 2 weeks	✓	*R*	*R*
5. *Invite them to attend a face-to-face meeting with other team members by setting up a Doodle schedule and sending it out.* Due date: 2 weeks	✓	*R*	*H*

How well did this plan work? Did you accomplish your goal?
Plan worked well, though some parts were harder than I expected and others were easier.

- **Were all of the steps needed?**

   Yes, definitely.

- **Were there additional steps that you did not anticipate? Which ones?**

   Not really.

- **Were the steps as hard as you anticipated?**

   —*It was harder than I thought to explain why I wanted a team . . . my draft was too long and too detailed. I needed the coach's help to edit it but still make it sound like me. But now I have a way to tell people who I am, what I need, and why I need it.*

   —*Doodle scheduling took a lot of time and troubleshooting, but now I know how to use it. Some people needed a nudge to fill it out; that took time.*

- **Would you do anything differently next time?**

   —*Nothing really. But next time I need to plan something, it will be easier.*

   —*But I would also allow more time for people to respond.*

   —*Now I know how to explain my situation, which is really helpful.*

FIGURE 7.2. A sample of how to create a team using the Action-Planning Form (Form 4.6).

In team meetings, students can see self-advocacy being modeled and can practice it themselves. Together, students and coaches can set an agenda for the first team meeting, and students can play as large a role in leading it as they feel comfortable. Typically, students play a larger role in running their own team meetings as their self-efficacy becomes stronger and their executive skills improve to where, eventually, they plan and run the team meeting themselves (Mazzotti, Kelley, & Coco, 2015). Regardless of the size of the role the student plays in the team meeting, reflecting on what worked well and what did not will activate self-regulated learning. Coaches may find the Strategy Usefulness and Next Steps form (Form 4.5) a helpful guide for this discussion.

Consider another situation that requires self-advocacy: figuring out what to do when accommodations are not being implemented. The following comments are typically made by students when this occurs.

> "It's hit or miss whether I get the slides before the lecture, but its fine, really, I don't want to get the TA in trouble."

> "I have preferred seating toward the front the class, but there's a group of students who get there early and take my seat. I don't know what to do."

> "I asked the instructor how to get additional time to take a quiz when it's in the middle of class, but he said that was not possible. I took the quiz with everyone else and blew it. Think I got a 4 out of 10 points."

> "I was supposed to take the exam in a quiet room in the department's building, but the instructor forgot and I ended up taking it with everyone else. My anxiety was through the roof."

When coaches ask students what they can do when these situations arise, the responses differ and depend in part on students' coping strategies (planners versus avoiders), their self-perception, and their communication skills. Some students want to discuss their options, make a decision on a course of action, and then follow through with it themselves, whereas other students are uncomfortable with approaching the instructor or TA and prefer to go through their disability specialist. The following scenario makes this point.

A student with a TBI, who suffered from anxiety and low self-esteem after being injured, also had executive function problems with planning, staying organized, and remembering new material. Her anxiety made all these problems worse. Her primary concern and *goal* was to do as well as she could in her classes, which meant she had to keep up-to-date with reviewing lecture material, itself a *self-regulation goal*. One of her accommodations (*a strategy solution*) was to receive and review lecture notes before class, but the instructor did not get the lecture notes to her for 2 consecutive weeks. After the second week she asked the instructor about not receiving the notes, even though she was extremely nervous doing so, saying "Dr. Smith, you remember me, right, that I'm the one that needs your lecture notes? I know you are really busy, but I really do need to get those." He said he would send them to her. Still, she did not receive the notes before the next two subsequent classes. At this point, she became anxious and nervous about now falling behind and became frustrated with the instructor's lack of follow-through. With coaching support, she decided to ask her disability specialist to contact the instructor. It is worth pointing out here that the student could have handled this differently, such as drafting another script or email to the instructor rather than approach the disability specialist. But because she had already spoken with the instructor, because she was very anxious, and because she was falling further behind, this was a timely solution. As soon as the student's disability specialist contacted the instructor, she received lecture notes for the next class and the remainder of the semester. The student was very relieved and her anxiety subsided. Removing the "stressor" for this student gave her enough confidence to get through a challenging course. In retrospect, she believed that she had acted appropriately; for her, the anxiety about having to remind instructors of her accommodations proved too great, and was a barrier in itself to her having equal access to materials that she needed. Prior to graduation, she answered the question "How useful were disability services to you?" from the CSS-BI as follows:

> "Whenever I had trouble with my instructors, my counselor would contact the instructor directly, so that was really convenient and helpful to me; I didn't have to worry. They also had me take exams over there [at the disability services center] so I didn't have to see how well prepared other students were, when I was not. I didn't have to deal with any of those emotions that just made studying and being in class even worse. So, yeah, my counselor was very helpful."

As is the case when coaching self-organization and self-learning, some students do not take advantage of or use their strategies. For the reasons described earlier in this chapter, not all students use their self-advocacy skills to access their accommodations. The following scenario involves a student who had sustained multiple concussions in high school and developed post-concussive symptoms that included being highly distractible and having chronic headaches and fatigue. His overall *goal* was to get good grades while managing his symptoms. One of his accommodations was to take exams in the distraction-free room at the disability services center. Again, this accommodation was a *strategy* intended to level the playing field for him. However, even with the coach's encouragement, he had been unwilling to do so, saying it was "such a hassle" and "more work than it's worth." While his performance on exams was acceptable to himself, his symptoms remained a problem. Then, after having a bad experience taking an exam in a so-called quiet room (provided by the instructor) where graduate students walked in and out to access the microwave, he created a plan to use the distraction-free room. His plan is illustrated in Figure 7.3. Notice that he anticipated that it would be "hard" to notify disability services when the exam was scheduled in order to reserve a quiet room and that taking the exam in a room provided by disability services would also be hard; these were his reasons for not taking advantage of this accommodation. However, his actual experience was different. The student made the following comments after using the distraction-free room to take the exam:

> STUDENT: It [distraction-free room] was so much better taking the exam there . . . but so funny, the distraction-free room has tons of distractions! There's a pencil sharpener, and the chair swivels around and back and forth. But I feel like I had way better posture almost because I was just so relaxed. So, I got comfortable, kicked back, and took the test (*large exhale*). I don't know how I did on it, but when I finished it was like "OK, I'm done." I didn't have a headache, didn't have to take a nap, nothing. I just had the rest of my day.
>
> COACH: Wow, I'm glad it went so well. This is a big change for you, huh?
>
> STUDENT: Yeah! I don't know how I did on the test, but I just felt so much better afterward.

Let's now turn to coaching students about how to self-advocate with peers and friends, where we must take into consideration the unexpected social challenges that students with executive function problems face in college. For example, individuals with TBI report having fewer friends than before their injury and that others, especially peers, do not seem to understand their problems (Kennedy et al., 2008, 2014). Additional factors, such as low self-esteem and difficulty adjusting to college, also likely play a role, as is the case for students with ADHD (Shaw-Zirt et al., 2005). Here are some comments based on follow-up questions from college student surveys.

> "I have fewer friends now; not everyone understands, they don't know how to be around me."
>
> "I can't tell if other people can tell that I had a brain injury. I don't walk with a limp and I have no visible scars."
>
> "They [my friends] don't get why I can't go out constantly. They don't understand that it takes me a long time to study if I want to get a good grade. It's not like high school—it's a lot harder and I need to study a lot more."
>
> "I once had someone say to me, 'Gee, I wish I could take a nap.'" (from a student with chronic fatigue from concussion in response to "Others don't understand my problems")

Goal: *To take my exam in the distraction-free room available at the disabilities services center in order to be more relaxed and have fewer postconcussion symptoms afterward.*

Steps in my plan	Done (✓)	E = easy; R = routine; H = hard	
		Will be . . .	Was
1. *Notify disability services when the exam is scheduled so a quiet room can be reserved.* Due date: 1 week ahead of exam	✓	*H*	*E*
2. *Let the instructor know I will be taking the exam there.* Due date: 1 week ahead of exam	✓	*E*	*E*
3. *Rearrange my schedule so that I can take the exam.* Due date: 1 week ahead of exam	✓	*R*	*R*
4. *Wear comfortable clothing.* Due date: day of exam	✓	*E*	*E*
5. *Take the exam.* Due date: same day that the rest of class takes the exam	✓	*H*	*E*

How well did this plan work? Did you accomplish your goal?
Really well! I didn't have a headache or have to go take a nap afterward.

- **Were all of the steps needed?**

  Yes.

- **Were there additional steps that you did not anticipate? Which ones?**

  No.

- **Were the steps as hard as you anticipated?**

  Not as hard.

- **Would you do anything differently next time?**

  Take my exams in the disability services center.

FIGURE 7.3. Taking an exam in the disability services center using the Action-Planning Form (Form 4.6).

Acquiring and maintaining relationships can be problematic for students with executive function problems because of their challenges with staying organized, prioritizing, creating and following through with plans, and forgetting appointments, among others. However, their social skills may hurt their relationships as well. Students who are disinhibited may talk before they think. Students who are unaware of the context, do not notice body language, or do not understand conversational signals may not adjust their communication accordingly. There is a rich literature on the social communication skills and therapeutic interventions that can help individuals with TBI that are beyond the scope of this text. Readers are referred to McDonald, Togher, and Code (2014) for an in-depth discussion of these issues.

For students who choose to address maintaining or establishing relationships with peers as a *goal,* having a plan that includes strategies that they themselves have chosen to implement will be crucial. Table 7.3 provides samples of self-advocacy communication strategies and the kinds of communication issues for which these strategies are well suited.

What strategies will be used and what the plan will look like depend on the student and his or her self-advocacy needs. To add a further complication, any plan will need to incorporate the other two domains of self-learning and self-management. For example, when students are unable to participate in activities with their peers, they may need to have scripts in place to explain their absence, coupled with suggestions of alternative plans. Developing scripts and brainstorming alternative plans can tax executive functions if students struggle to think flexibly

TABLE 7.3. Self-Advocacy Communication Strategies for College Students with Executive Function Problems

Strategy	Useful for students who . . .
Observe–wait–listen–speak (OWLS)	Are disinhibited in their communication, monopolize conversations, or tend to talk without paying attention to the context.
Stop–think–accept–relax–reframe–solve (STARRS)	Struggle to know how to respond when others' responses are neutral or negative. Particularly useful for students were are nervous or anxious.
Who, what, when, where, and how	Have trouble anticipating and planning conversations they may have in academic and/or social situations.
Conversational scripts	Are unsure how to start conversations or are nervous about possible responses to which they in turn need to respond.
Summarizing and clarifying others' responses	Are unsure that they have understood; need additional time to consider how they will respond.
Positive self-talk	Are not confident in their social communication skills or who anticipate negative responses.

or generate ideas, and particularly if students have other memory, language, or attention deficits. The coach's role will be to provide guidance in these areas so that students can also address their self-advocacy needs. Similarly, if students struggle with time management, they may want to consider planning time for friends in a routinized fashion, such as Friday and Saturday evenings only or Wednesday and Sunday afternoons. Students can block these days off in their planners and know that these times are free to suggest to friends, rather than struggling in the moment to decide if they have other commitments in place.

When establishing relationships, students also may need to consider less-structured activities as *solutions or strategies* that can make them available to others in a way that allows for a more informal social connection. In the example that follows, the GSAA self-regulation process occurs continuously and naturally as the student was coached to explore and experience ways to achieve her *goal* of making new friends.

As a result of a brain injury, the student had executive function problems that included difficulty in generating ideas, especially solutions, and then putting those solutions into action. Initially, she appeared overwhelmed in college and responded by withdrawing and avoiding social situations. Instead, she focused solely on maintaining her grades. After a semester of being socially isolated, she realized she had not made any new friends. Her roommates often spent time together without her. She was naturally shy, used avoidance as a coping mechanism, and was unsure what to say when meeting strangers or, in the case of her roommates, people she did know well. With the assistance of the coach, she identified situations as steps in a plan that could result in conversations, and made a plan as to *when and how* she could spend more time with her peers. Her overall *performance goal* was to expand her social circle, but her *self-regulation goals* were targeted toward meeting the *steps in the plan* (e.g., eating in the common areas with her roommates instead of retreating to her room) and meeting other students in her classes by coming early and staying a few minutes after class. Additionally, since she had participated in chorus in high school before her brain injury, she expanded her extracurricular activities to include chorus as a logical way to extend her social circle. Thus, the *steps in her plan became her strategies* that she would implement to attempt to make new friends.

She and the coach developed a goal-attainment scale (GAS; Chapter 5) so that she could track her progress on the three components that would lead to making new friends. Using three separate GASs, her target goals were to (1) eat at least half of her meals with her roommates, (2) talk to at least two students each week before or after class (or during group discussions if that occurred), and (3) join choir and meet at least three students during the first week of rehearsal. At first the student was concerned that these steps might be too demanding, but found it was easier than she had expected because she implemented (*act*) the plan at the beginning of the semester, a time when many students are open to making new friends. Although the GASs were not designed to measure whether the connections she made developed into long-term friendships, it was an important confidence booster for her to be able to introduce herself and have conversations with unfamiliar students. She also found that because her roommates had developed strong friendships among themselves, she did not have to lead conversations during meals or when watching a show on Netflix with them in the evening. Instead, by including herself as a part of these activities, she was able to slowly get to know them better and they her as well. She found that the plan was working well and as she had more experiences meeting peers, she began to readjust her perception of herself—that she was not really as shy as she thought when there was a common activity or interest that made these initial contacts easier. Therefore, she did not *adjust* the plan, and in the end made new friends. This doesn't mean it was always easy. There were times when she withdrew and avoided people, but with coaching, she learned that this typically occurred when she was overwhelmed with her study workload and that it was short-lived. Thus, her self-awareness of her own social behavior increased tremendously throughout this process, and her self-confidence grew such that she knew, in the future, she would have little trouble in being able to make friends.

A final comment is warranted about coaching self-advocacy in college students with executive function problems. Not all students want or even need to be coached in self-advocacy. Typically these students need coaching for self-organization and self-learning, but for a variety of reasons, do not see the need for coaching support in self-advocacy. We have observed two kinds of student scenarios wherein self-advocacy was not addressed.

The first scenario applies to students who are more independent than others and who need little support in this area. They are more mature in their own self-determination, and know what they want from college and how they are going to get it. Usually these students are getting coached on self-organization and self-learning, but have a wait-and-see attitude about getting any self-advocacy support. For example, one of our students insisted that he had very few impairments after being injured and, while his unwillingness to explicitly acknowledge that his deficits were a challenge for coaches at times, he was willing to be coached in these two domains, and he used his accommodations as needed. In retrospect, we realized that he had abilities that made him a strong self-advocate: he was an independent decision maker who seldom relied on his family even before his injury, he had a determined career path, he had excellent verbal communication skills, and he had an outgoing and friendly personality.

This second scenario is more common than the one just described. Although all students with executive function problems need self-advocacy skills for working with college staff, not all students want or need self-advocacy support with friends. Of the students that we have coached, the first and foremost priority was to succeed academically; later, once they had experienced some academic success and realized that they were going to be able to get through college, only then did they give their social life much attention. For these students, self-advocacy with friends and peers became a priority later in college, and they may have relied more on family and old friends. However, this also means, that when they are ready to become a better advocate with friends, they are doing so with a more positive self-perception and self-image of who they are as a person; that they are individuals with many strengths and few disabilities. Having these thoughts about themselves can help them make better choices later about whom *they choose* as friends.

ADDITIONAL RESOURCES

- The book *Accommodations in Higher Education under the Americans with Disabilities Act (ADA): A No-Nonsense Guide for Clinicians, Educators, Administrators, and Lawyers* (Gordon & Keiser, 2000).
- "A Practical Guide for People with Disabilities Who Want to Go to College": *http://tucollaborative.org/pdfs/education/College_Guide.pdf.*
- "Making Accessibility Decisions for ALL Students": *www.cehd.umn.edu/NCEO/OnlinePubs/briefs/brief11/brief11.html.*
- Self-advocacy training and educational resources include the following:
  - "ME! Lessons for Teaching Self-Awareness & Self-Advocacy": *www.ou.edu/education/centers-and-partnerships/zarrow/trasition-education-materials/me-lessons-for-teaching-self-awareness-and-self-advocacy.html.*
  - Teaching self-advocacy skills to students: *https://teachingselfadvocacy.wordpress.com.*
  - Priority | Best Practices in Self-Advocacy Skill Building: *www.parentcenterhub.org/repository/priority-selfadvocacy.*
  - National Gateway to Self-Determination: *http://ngsd.org/audience-topic/for-people-with-disabilities/self-advocacy.*

Team Members

My team members are people I can go to for support or assistance.

Name	Relationship	What will they do?	Contact information
Whom can I go to for . . . ?			
Whom can I go to for . . . ?			
Whom can I go to for . . . ?			
Whom can I go to for . . . ?			

CHAPTER 8

Coaching toward Independence

The final phase of coaching involves making the final transition from yourself as coach to empowering the student to be his or her own coach. Your ultimate aim is to enable students to self-coach. The objectives of this concluding chapter are the following:

- To describe tools that students can use to help them coach themselves.
- To help readers consider how to translate dynamic coaching into their practice of supporting students with executive function problems.

TOOLS THAT FOSTER SELF-COACHING

The final step toward student self-coaching is not as hard as it may seem if you, as a coach, adhered to the principles and the approach provided in this book. By now you know that coaching self-regulation entails some explicit instruction, while at the same time working with students to give them control over setting goals, proposing strategies and solutions, and implementing and adjusting an action plan along the way. The transition to self-coaching is a natural progression toward independence, which students should not experience as a sudden change. Some suggested ways to accomplish this are below.

First, *students' self-reflection* at the end of each semester and academic year are a way to demonstrate how much they have accomplished, how much they have learned about themselves, and how the knowledge and skills they have acquired can be used in other situations. Student-based outcomes (i.e, tangible accomplishments) can include but are not limited to improved grades on assignments and in courses; positive outcomes should reflect the independence students gain by making larger decisions about an academic major and a career path. Regardless, it is important not only to review what students accomplished, but also to discuss how their self-regulation allowed them to achieve their goals. For example, a discussion with students about the areas they found more or less challenging than they thought can help to shape their sense of self and their self-efficacy (e.g., Form 4.2, Self-Reflection: Start and Form 4.3, Self-Reflection: End). And as we know, students with disabilities need a strong sense of self-efficacy to be successful at college and at work. At this time, coaches and students should explicitly discuss that now the student knows how to:

- Identify and modify solutions and strategies to accommodate their needs, abilities, and disabilities.
- Assess his or her own ability to implement strategies, including being more aware of what is challenging and what is easier or more routine.
- Rely on others for support, ranging from disability services to friends and family.
- Become more resilient by revisiting and adjusting a strategy or a goal.
- Establish positive organizational, studying, and self-advocacy routines.

Second, *portfolios* are very useful tools for helping students keep track of all of the strategies and solutions they have learned while being coached. Portfolios are particularly useful for students who have the executive function problems of planning, organizing, remembering, and learning. Portfolios are a single place in which students can record not only what they have accomplished (e.g., grades in courses), but also what strategies worked, when they worked, how hard (or easy) they were to use, and additional uses of strategies. Form 4.7, Student Summary of Strategies, can be included in the portfolio to remind students of the strategies they learned to use and how these strategies could be used for other activities. Having students start a portfolio in the first semester of coaching and updating it regularly enables them to keep an ongoing record of their performance and of what they have learned about themselves as well. Portfolios are typically organized by self-identified categories and can range from electronic ones (e.g., Evernote) to paper notebooks.

Coaches will find that their work is nearly finished when students are taking over the planning, strategizing, implementing, and adjusting themselves. As students become more comfortable with self-regulating, coaches will have little to do other than listen and lend positive feedback. An indication of this is the need for fewer coaching sessions across semesters. Still, many students need to review their plan with the coach at the beginning of the next semester or academic year. These meetings simply serve to remind the student of the planning, organizing, studying, and self-advocacy routines they had learned while being coached. Having a portfolio helps remind students of their previously established routines and is used to facilitate the discussions at these meetings.

Finally, it is worth remembering that when coaching students who get "stuck" it is helpful to revisit the stages of change by Prochaska and colleagues (1992) and expanded upon by Di Clemente and Velasquez (2002), as well as the coaching suggestions found in Table 4.1. Revisiting these stages of change will remind coaches of other approaches besides the ones they have already used. But keep in mind that for some problems, such as clinical depression, anxiety, or compulsive behavior, students are best referred to a mental health professional. Depending on the coach's disciplinary background and scope of practice, she or he may be trained to assess and provide therapeutic support. For example, as a speech–language pathologist, I do not provide psychotherapy to students for depression, anxiety, or other mental issues, yet I can provide more extensive intervention such as cognitive rehabilitation and speech–language therapy, which are within my scope of practice. When the nature of the problem is beyond a coach's scope of practice, however, it's time to refer the student to a professional who is trained and licensed to help.

INTEGRATING DYNAMIC COACHING INTO YOUR PRACTICE

Now that you have learned about executive functions, self-regulation, and dynamic coaching, it's time to consider how this approach will be integrated into your clinical or educational practice. You may have some lingering questions, such as the ones that follow.

Which parts of dynamic coaching am I certain I understand, and which parts am I less certain I understand?

Your answer to this question may depend on the discipline you were trained in. For example, speech–language pathologists and occupational therapists may be confident in identifying strategies based on their background in cognitive rehabilitation, whereas psychologists may be confident in using MI techniques to facilitate discussions. Consider finding colleagues from both within *and* outside your discipline with whom you can meet and discuss those areas that you are less certain about. Most likely, you will find that other colleagues will be able to provide additional explanations or examples from their own practice to assist you, and that you will be able to do the same for them.

Are the students I work with good candidates for this approach?

Students who have executive function problems along with mild to moderate attention, memory, and learning impairments are good candidates for this approach. Students with more severe cognitive impairments will likely need more intensive, didactic approaches and may not be good candidates.

Am I in an environment where I can work with students who are currently in college?

If you are a rehabilitation professional who works with outpatients, you can certainly coach students with ABI who are currently enrolled in college. While it is preferable to be working on a college campus, this may not be possible; the alternative is to provide coaching as an outpatient service. On-campus clinics, such as campus study skill centers, disability service centers, and speech-language clinics, are ideal environments for coaching students.

Are there discipline-related barriers in place that could prevent me from using this approach? What are those barriers and how can they be managed?

Coaches must consider their discipline-specific knowledge and skills in order to practice. Rehabilitation professionals (speech–language pathologists, occupational therapists, psychologists, vocational rehabilitation counselors) work in disciplines that have clear practice guidelines and scopes of practice. For example, the practice in each of these disciplines includes cognitive rehabilitation therapy (CRT) for individuals with ABI; the dynamic coaching described in this book is indeed an extension of CRT applied to supporting college students with executive function problems. Although these disciplines have much in common, they do emphasize different aspects of human behavior. For example, if a coach who is a vocational rehabilitation counselor realizes that the student needs direct instruction to address reading issues, then a referral to a speech–language pathologist is in order. If a coach who is a speech–language pathologist realizes that the student is ready to explore vocations, then the student should be referred to a vocational counselor. If a coach who is a college disability specialist suspects that the student needs treatment for clinical depression, then a counselor or mental health professional should be consulted.

Can I bill for coaching services?

The short answer is yes. For coaches who need to bill for their services, coaching, like other forms of CRT, speech–language therapy, and occupational therapy, is billable as long as goals are measurable and functional. Our coaching services at the University of Minnesota were billed through a contract with the Minnesota Department of Employment and Economic Development (DEED).

In closing, remember that learning to use dynamic coaching is similar to what we are asking of our college students, except that we can rely on having strong executive functions. You'll find that some coaching skills come easy to you and others are more challenging, and you'll end up modifying the coaching goals you set for yourself or modifying the strategies if they don't work. But be resilient, and realize that when learning something new, it doesn't always turn out like you thought it would. Remember that you have a partner in this endeavor too, your student, and oftentimes the solutions and outcomes that emerge from this partnership turn out to be better than either of you could have imagined alone.

References

Adams, C. (2013, March, 14). Millions went to war in Iraq, Afghanistan leaving life-long scars. Retrieved from *www.mcclatchydc.com/news/nation-world/national/article24746680.html*.

Allen, C. C., & Ruff, R. M. (1990). Self-rating versus neuropsychological performance of moderate versus severe head-injured patients. *Brain Injury, 4*(1), 7–17.

Alves, W., Macciocchi, S. N., & Barth, J. T., (1993). Postconcussive symptoms after uncomplicated mild head injury. *Journal of Head Trauma Rehabilitation, 8*(3), 48–59.

American Psychiatric Association. (1980). *Diagnostic and statistical manual of mental disorders* (3rd ed.). Washington, DC: Author.

American Psychiatric Association. (2000). *Diagnostic and statistical manual of mental disorders* (4th ed., text revision). Washington, DC: Author.

American Psychiatric Association. (2013). *Diagnostic and statistical manual of mental disorders* (5th ed.). Arlington, VA: Author.

Anson, K., & Ponsford, J. (2006) Evaluation of a coping skills group following traumatic brain injury. *Brain Injury, 20*(2), 167–178.

Association on Higher Education and Disability. (2000). Guidelines for documentation of a learning disability in adolescents and adults. Retrieved from *www.ahead.org.*

Bandura, A. (1997). *Self-efficacy: The exercise of control.* New York: Freeman.

Banks, S., & Dinges, D. F. (2007). Behavioral and physiological consequences of sleep restriction. *Journal of Clinical Sleep Medicine, 3*(5), 518–528.

Barkley, R. A. (1990). *Attention-deficit hyperactivity disorder: A handbook for diagnosis and treatment.* New York: Guilford Press.

Barkley, R. A. (1997). *ADHD and the nature of self-control.* New York: Guilford Press.

Barnea-Goraly, N., Menon, V., Eckert, M., Tamm, L., Bammer, R., Karchemskiy, A., et al. (2005). White matter development during childhood and adolescence: A cross-sectional diffusion tensor imaging study. *Cerebral Cortex, 15*(12), 1848–1854.

Beauchamp, H., & Kiewra, K. R. (2004). Assessment of career maturity and self- advocacy skills. In E. M. Levinson (Ed.), *Transition from school to post-school life for individuals with disabilities: Assessment from an educational and school psychological perspective* (pp. 150–188). Springfield, IL: Charles C Thomas.

Belanger, H. G., Donnell, A. J., & Vanderploeg, R. D. (2014). Special issues with mild TBI in veterans and active duty service members. In M. Sherer & A. M. Sander (Eds.), *Handbook on the neuropsychology of traumatic brain injury* (pp. 389–412). New York: Springer.

Ben-Eliyahu, A., & Bernacki, M. L. (2015). Addressing complexities in self-regulated learning: A focus on contextual factors, contingencies, and dynamic relations. *Metacognition and Learning, 10*(1), 1–13.

Berger, B. A., & Villaume, W. A. (2013). *Motivational interviewing for health care professionals: A sensible approach.* Washington, DC: American Pharmacists Association.

Bjork, E. L., & Bjork, R. A. (2011). Making things hard on yourself, but in a good way: Creating desirable difficulties to enhance learning. In M. A. Gernsbacher, R. W. Pew, L. M. Hough, & J. R. Pomerantz (Eds.), *Psychology and the real world: Essays illustrating fundamental contributions to society* (pp. 56–64). New York: Worth.

Bombardier, C. H., & Rimmele, C. T. (1999). Motivational interviewing to prevent alcohol abuse after traumatic brain injury: A case series. *Rehabilitation Psychology, 44*(1), 52–67.

Borkum, J. M. (2007). Headache nosology and warning signs. In *Chronic headaches: Biology, psychology, and behavioral treatment* (pp. 3–24). Mahwah, NJ: Erlbaum.

Boyer, B. E., Geurts, H. M., Prins, P. J. M., & Van der Oord, S. (2014). Two novel CBTs for adolescents with ADHD: The value of planning skills. *European Child and Adolescent Psychiatry, 24*(9), 1075–1090.

Brady, J., Busse, R. T., & Lopez, C. J. (2014). Monitoring school consultation intervention outomes for data-based decision making: An application of the goal attainment scaling method. *Counseling Outcome Research and Evaluation, 5*(1), 64–70.

Branscum, P., & Sharma, M. (2010). A review of motivational interviewing-based interventions targeting problematic drinking among college students. *Alcoholism Treatment Quarterly, 28*(1), 63–77.

Brown, B. (2010). *The gifts of imperfection.* Center City, MN: Hazelden.

Brown, J. I., Fishco, V. V., & Hanna, G. (1993). *The Nelson–Denny reading test.* Itasca, IL: Riverside.

Brush, J., & Camp, C. (1998). Using spaced retrieval as an intervention during speech-language therapy. *Clinical Gerontology, 19,* 51–64.

Busch, R. M., McBride, A., Curtiss, G., & Vanderploeg, R. D. (2005). The components of executive functioning in traumatic brain injury. *Journal of Clinical and Experimental Neuropsychology, 27*(8), 1022–1032.

Butler, D. L. (1995). Promoting strategic learning by post secondary students with learning disabilities. *Journal of Learning Disabilities, 28,* 170–190.

Carver, C. S., & Scheier, M. F. (1991). Self-regulation and the self. In J. Strauss & G. R. Goethals (Eds.), *The self: Interdisciplinary approaches* (pp. 168–207). New York: Springer-Verlag.

Carver, C. S., & Scheier, M. F. (2001). Self-regulatory perspectives on personality. In T. Millon & M. J. Lerner (Eds.), *Handbook of psychology* (pp. 185–208). Hoboken, NJ: Wiley.

Castro, C. A. (2006). Battlemind training I: Transitioning from combat to home. Retrieved June 20, 2015, from *www.ptsd.ne.gov/pdfs/WRAIR-battlemind-training-Brochure.pdf.*

Centers for Disease Control, National Institutes of Health, Department of Defense, &

Department of Veterans Affairs Leadership Panel. (2013). Report to Congress on traumatic brain injury in the United States: Understanding the public health problem among current and former military personnel. Retrieved November 8, 2016, from *www.cdc.gov/traumaticbraininjury/pdf/report_to_congress_on_traumatic_brain_injury_2013-a.pdf.*

Charles, C., Gafni, A., & Whelan, T. (1999). Shared decision making in the physician–patient encounter: Revisiting the shared treatment decision-making model. *Social Sciences and Medicine, 49,* 651–661.

Cicerone, K. D., Dahlberg, C., Kalmar, K., Langenbahn, D. M., Malec, J. F., Bergquist, T. F., et al. (2000). Evidence-based cognitive rehabilitation: Recommendation for clinical practice. *Archives of Physical Medicine and Rehabilitation, 81*(12), 1596–1615.

Cicerone, K. D., Langenbahn, D. M., Braden, C., Malec, J. F., Kalmar, K., Fraas, M. et al. (2011). Evidence-based cognitive rehabilitation: Updated review of the literature from 2003 through 2008. *Archives of Physical Medicine and Rehabilitation, 92*(4), 519–530.

Cicerone, K. D., & Wood, J. C. (1987). Planning disorder after closed head injury: A case study. *Archives of Physical Medicine and Rehabilitation, 68,* 111–115.

Cifu, D. X., & Blake, C. (2011). *Overcoming post-deployment syndrome: A six-step mission to health.* New York: Springer.

Coll, J. E., Weiss, E. L., & Yarvis J. S. (2010). No one leaves unchanged: Insights for civilian mental health care professionals into the military experience and culture. *Social Work in Health Care, 50*(7), 487–500.

Constantinidou, F., & Kennedy, M. R. T (2017). Traumatic brain injury. In I. Papathanasiou, P. Coppens, & C. Potagas (Eds.), *Aphasia and related disorders* (2nd ed., pp. 421–454). Burlington, MA: Jones & Bartlett.

Cory, R. C. (2011). Disability services offices for students with disabilities: A campus resource. *New Directions for Higher Education, 2011*(154), 27–36.

Covassin, T., Stearne, D., & Elbin, R. (2008). Concussion history and postconcussion neurocognitive performance and symptoms in collegiate athletes. *Journal of Athletic Training, 43*(2), 119–124.

Dawson, D. R., Cantanzaro, A. M., Firestone, J., Schwartz, M., & Stuss, D. T. (2006). Changes in coping style following traumatic brain injury and their relationship to productivity status. *Brain and Cognition, 60*(2), 214–216.

Dawson, P., & Guare, R. (2012). *Coaching students with executive skills deficits.* New York: Guilford Press.

DeBaca, C. (2010). Resiliency and academic performance. Retrieved from *www.scholarcentric.com/wp-content/uploads/2014/03/SC_Resiliency_Academic_Performance_WP.pdf.*

Defense and Veterans Brain Injury Center. (2015, February 23). DoD worldwide numbers for traumatic brain injury. Retrieved from *www.dvbic.org/TBI-Numbers.*

Delis, D. C., Kaplan, E., & Kramer, J. H. (2001). *Delis–Kaplan Executive Function System.* San Antonio, TX: Pearson Education.

Demiroren, M., Turan, S., & Oztuna, D. (2016). Medical students' self-efficacy in problem-based learning and its relationship with self-regulated learning. *Medical Education Online, 21.* [Epub ahead of print]

DiClemente, C. C., & Velasquez, M. M. (2002). Motivational interviewing and the stages of change. In W. R. Miller & S. Rollnick *Motivational interviewing: Preparing people for change* (2nd ed., pp. 201–216). New York: Guilford Press.

Donders, J., & Strong, C. A. (2016). Latent structure of the Behavior Rating Inventory of Executive Function—Adult Version (BRIEF-A) after mild traumatic brain injury. *Archives of Clinical Neuropsychology, 31,* 29–36.

Drake, A. I., Gray, N., Yoder, S., Pramuka, M., & Llewellyn, M. (2000). Factors predicting return to work following mild traumatic brain injury: A discriminant analysis. *Journal of Head Trauma Rehabilitation, 15*(5), 1103–1112.

Draper, K., & Ponsford, J. (2008). Cognitive functioning ten years following traumatic brain injury and rehabilitation. *Neuropsychology, 22*(5), 618–625.

Dunivin, K. O. (1994). Military culture: Change and continuity. *Armed Forces and Society, 20*(4), 531–547.

Dunlosky, J., Hertzog, C., Kennedy, M., & Thiede, K. (2005). The self-monitoring approach for effective learning. *Cognitive Technology, 10,* 4–11.

Dunning, D., Johnson, K., Ehrlinger, J., & Kruger, J. (2003). Why people fail to recognize their own incompetence. *Current Directions in Psychological Science, 12*(3), 83–87.

DuPaul, G. J., Schaughency, E. A., Weyandt, L. L., Tripp, G., Kiesner, J., Ota, K., et al. (2001). Self-report of ADHD symptoms in university students: Cross-gender and cross-national prevalence. *Journal of Learning Disabilities, 34,* 370–379.

DuPaul, G. J., Weyandt, L. L., O'Dell, S. M., & Varejao, M. (2009). College students with ADHD: Current status and future directions. *Journal of Attention Disorders, 13*(3), 234–250.

Ehlhardt, L., Sohlberg, M. M., Kennedy, M., Coelho, C., Ylvisaker, M., & Turkstra, L. (2008). Evidence-based practice guidelines for instructing individuals with neurogenic memory impairments: What have we learned in the past 20 years? *Neuropsychological Rehabilitation, 18*(3), 300–342.

Ellison, M. L., Mueller, L., Smelson, D., Corrigan, P. W., Terres-Stone, R. A., Bokhour, B. G., et al. (2012). Supporting the education goals of post-9.11 veterans with self-reported PTSD symptoms. *Psychiatric Rehabilitation Journal, 35*(3), 209–217.

Evans, C. J., Kirby, J. R., & Fabrigar, L. R. (2003). Approaches to learning, need for cognition, and strategic flexibility among university students. *Journal of Educational Psychology, 73*(4), 507–528.

Exum, H. A., Coll, J. E., & Weiss, E. L. (2011). *A civilian counselor's primer for counseling veterans.* Deer Park, NY: Linus.

Field, S., Martin, J., Miller, R., Ward, M., & Wehmeyer, M. (1998). Self-determination for persons with disabilities: A position statement of the division on career development and transition. *Career Development for Exceptional Individuals, 21*(2), 113–128.

Field, S., Parker, D. R., Sawilowsky, S., & Rolands, L. (2010). *College well-being scale.* Detroit, MI: Wayne State University College of Education.

Field, S., Parker, D. R., Sawilowsky, S., & Rolands, I. (2013). Assessing the impact of ADHD coaching services on university students' learning skills, self-regulation, and well-being. *Journal of Postsecondary Education and Disability, 26*(1), 67–81.

Finn, D., Getzel, E. E., & McManus, S. (2008). Adapting the self-determined learning model for instruction of college students with disabilities. *Career Development for Exceptional Individuals, 31*(2), 85–93.

Flavell, J. H. (1979). Metacognition and cognitive monitoring: A new area of cognitive-developmental inquiry. *American Psychologist, 34*(10), 906–911.

Folkman, S., & Lazarus, R. (1988). *Ways of Coping Questionnaire manual.* Palto Alto, CA: Consulting Psychologists Press.

Gehrman, P., Seelig, A., Jacobson, I., Boyko, E., Hooper, T., & Gackstetter, G. (2013). Predeployment sleep duration and insomnia symptoms as risk factors for new-onset mental health disorders following military deployment. *Sleep, 36,* 1009–1018.

Getzel, E. E., & Thoma, C. A. (2008). Experiences of college students with disabilities and the importance of self-determination in higher education settings. *Career Development for Exceptional Individuals, 31*(2), 77–84.

Giacino, J. T., & Cicerone, K. D. (1998). Varieties of deficit unawareness after brain injury. *Journal of Head Trauma Rehabilitation, 13,* 1–15.

Gioia, G. A., Isquith, P. K., Guy, S. C., & Kenworthy, L. (2002). Confirmatory factor analysis of the Behavior Rating Inventory of Executive Function (BRIEF) in a clinical sample. *Child Neuropsychology, 8*(4), 249–257.

Gordon, M., & Keiser, S. (Eds.). (2000). *Accommodations in higher education under the Americans with Disabilities Act (ADA): A no-nonsense guide for clinicians, educators, administrators, and lawyers.* New York: Guilford Press.

Graham, D. P., & Cardon, A. L. (2008). An update of substance use and treatment following traumatic brain injury. *Annals of the New York Academy of Sciences, 11*(41), 148–162.

Grossman, P. D. (2009). Foreword with a challenge: Leading our campuses away from the perfect storm. *Journal of Postsecondary Education and Disability, 22*(1), 4–8.

Gunstad, J., & Suhr, J. A. (2001). "Expectation as etiology" versus "the good old days": Postconcussion syndrome symptom reporting in athletes, headache sufferers, and depressed individuals. *Journal of the International Neuropsychological Society, 7*(3), 323–333.

Gunstad, J., & Suhr, J. A. (2004). Cognitive factors in postconcussion syndrome symptom report. *Archives of Clinical Neuropsychology, 19*(3), 391–405.

Halstead, M. E., McAvoy, K., Devore, C. D., Carl, R., Lee, M., & Logan, K. (2013). Returning to learning following a concussion. *Pediatrics, 132*(5), 948–957.

Hart, T., & Evans, J. (2006). Self-regulation and goal theories in brain injury rehabilitation. *Journal of Head Trauma and Rehabilitation, 21*(2), 142–155.

Hartman-Hall, H. M., & Haaga, D. A. F. (2002). College students' willingness to seek help for their learning disabilities. *Learning Disability Quarterly, 25,* 263–274.

Haskins, E. C., Cicerone, K., Dams-O'Connor, K., Eberle, R., Langenbahn, D., & Shapiro-Rosenbaum, A. (2012). *Cognitive rehabilitation manual: Translating evidence-based recommendations into practice.* Reston, VA: American Congress of Rehabilitation Medicine.

Herrero, D. (2014). The relationship among achievement motivation, hope, and resilience and their effects on academic achievement among first-year college students enrolled in a Hispanic-serving institution. Retrieved from *http://hdl.handle.net/1969.6/601.*

Hersh, D., Worral, L., Howe, T., Sherratt, S., & Davidson, B. (2012). SMARTER goal setting in aphasic rehabilitation. *Aphasiology, 26*(2), 220–233.

Hoffman, W., Schmeichel, B. J., & Baddeley, A. D. (2012). Executive functions and self-regulation. *Trends in Cognitive Sciences, 16*(3), 174–180.

Hoge, C. W. (2010). *Once a warrior always a warrior: Navigating the transition from combat to home including combat stress, PTSD, and mTBI.* Guilford, CT: Lyons Press.

Hoge, C. W., Castro, C. A., Messer, S. C., McGurk, D., Cotting, D. I., & Koffman, R. L. (2004). Combat duty in Iraq and Afghanistan, mental health problems, and barriers to care. *New England Journal of Medicine, 351*(1), 13–22.

Hoge, C. W., Goldberb, H. M., & Castro, C. A. (2009). Care of war veterans with mild traumatic brain injury: Flawed perspectives. *New England Journal of Medicine, 360*(16), 1588–1591.

Hoge, C. W., McGurk, D., Thomas, J. L., Cox, A. L., Engel, C. C., & Castro, C. A. (2008). Mild traumatic brain injury in US soldiers returning from Iraq. *New England Journal of Medicine, 358*(5), 453–463.

Hooker, R. D. (2003). Soldiers of the state: Reconsidering American civil–military relations: Parameters. *U.S. Army War College Quarterly, 33*(4), 4–18.

Hsieh, M., Ponsford, J., Wong, D., & McKay, A. (2012). Exploring variables associated with change in cognitive behaviour therapy (CBT) for anxiety following traumatic brain injury. *Disability and Rehabilitation, 34*(5), 408–415.

Hunt, A., Le Dorze, G., Polatojko, H., Bottari, C., & Dawson, D. R. (2015). Communication during goal-setting in brain injury rehabilitation: What helps and what hinders? *British Journal of Occupational Therapy, 78*(8), 488–498.

Hux, K., Bush, E., Zickefoose, S., Holmberg, M., Henderson, A., & Simanek G. (2010). Exploring the study skills and accommodations used by college student survivors of traumatic brain injury. *Brain Injury, 24*, 13–26.

Institute of Medicine. (2011). *Cognitive rehabilitation therapy for traumatic brain injury.* Washington, DC: Author.

Iverson, G. L. (2005). Outcome from mild traumatic brain injury. *Current Opinion in Psychiatry: Neuropsychiatry, 18*(3), 301–317.

Iverson, G. L. (2006). Misdiagnosis of the persistent postconcussion syndrome in patients with depression. *Archives of Clinical Neuropsychology, 21*(4), 303–310.

Iverson, G. L. (2010). Clinical and methodological challenges with assessing mild traumatic brain injury in the military. *Journal of Head Trauma Rehabilitation, 25*(5), 313–319.

Iverson, G. L., Gaetz, M., Lovell, M., & Collins, M. (2004). Relation between subjective fogginess and neuropsychological testing following concussion. *Journal of International Neuropsychology Society, 10* 1–3.

Iverson, G. L., Langlois, J. A., McCrea, M. A., & Kelly, J. P. (2009). Challenges associated with post-deployment screening for mild traumatic brain injury in military personnel. *The Clinical Neuropsychologist, 23*(8), 1299–1314.

Janiga, S. J., & Costenbader, V. (2002). The transition from high school to postsecondary education for students with learning disabilities: A survey of college service coordinators. *Journal of Learning Disabilities, 35*, 163–172.

Jelinek, P. A. (2014, March, 24). Half of veterans on G.I. Bill graduate, report estimates. Retrieved from *www.huffingtonpost.com/2014/03/24/veterans-gi-bill_n_5019385.html*.

Jowkar, B., Kojuri, J., Kohoulat, N., & Hayat, A. A. (2014). Academic resilience in education: The role of achievement goal orientations. *Journal of Advances in Medical Education and Professionalism, 2*(1), 33–38.

Kadzikowska-Wrzosek, R. (2012). Perceived stress, emotional ill-being and psychosomatic symptoms in high school students: The moderating effect of self-regulation competences. *Psychiatry and Psychotherapy, 14*(3), 25–33.

Kahneman, D., & Tversky, A. (1979). Intuitive prediction: Biases and corrective procedures. *TIMS Studies in Management Science, 12,* 313–327.

Katon, W., Berg, A. O., Robins, A. J., & Risse, S. (1986). Depression: Medical utilization and somatization. *Western Journal of Medicine, 144*(5), 564–568.

Katon, W., Kleinman, A., & Rosen, G. (1982). Depression and somatization: A review, part two. *American Journal of Medicine, 72*(2), 241–247.

Kennedy, M. R. T. (2001). Retrospective confidence judgments made by adults with traumatic brain injury: Relative and absolute accuracy. *Brain Injury, 15,* 469–487.

Kennedy, M. R. T. (2014). Evidence-based practice and cognitive rehabilitation therapy. In S. McDonald, L. Togher, & C. Code (Eds.), *Social and communication disorders following traumatic brain injury* (2nd ed., pp. 282–306). New York: Psychology Press.

Kennedy, M. R. T. (2016). *The College Survey for Students with Other Disabilities* (CSS-OD). Orange, CA: Chapman University.

Kennedy, M. R. T., Carney, E., & Peters, S. M. (2003). Predictions of recall and study strategy decisions after brain injury. *Brain Injury, 17,* 1043–1064.

Kennedy, M. R. T., & Coelho, C. (2005). Self-regulation after traumatic brain injury: A framework for intervention of memory and problem solving. *Seminars in Speech and Language, 26*(4), 242–255.

Kennedy, M. R. T., Coelho, C., Turkstra, L., Ylvisaker, M., Sohlberg, M. M., Yorkston, K., et al. (2008). Intervention for executive functions after traumatic brain injury: A systematic review, meta-analysis and clinical recommendations. *Journal of Neuropsychology Rehabilitation, 18*(3), 257–299.

Kennedy, M. R. T., DeSalvio, G., & Nguyen, V. (2015). *College Survey for Students with Concussion and Other Injuries* (CSS-CO). Orange, CA: Chapman University.

Kennedy, M. R. T., & Krause, M. O. (2009). The College Survey for Students with Brain Injury (CSS-BI). Retrieved from *http://neurocognitivelab.com/wp-content/uploads/2011/12/College-Survey-for-Students-with-Brain-Injury.pdf.*

Kennedy, M. R. T., & Krause, M. O. (2011). Self-regulated learning in a dynamic coaching model for supporting college students with traumatic brain injury: Two case reports. *Journal of Head Trauma Rehabilitation, 26*(3), 212–223.

Kennedy, M. R. T., Krause, M. O., & O'Brien, K. (2014). Psychometric properties of the college survey for students with brain injury: Individuals with and without traumatic brain injury, *Brain Injury, 28*(13–14), 1748–1757.

Kennedy, M. R. T., Krause, M. O., & Turkstra, L. (2008). An electronic survey about college experiences after traumatic brain injury. *NeuroRehabilitation, 23*(6), 511–520.

Kennedy, M. R. T., O'Brien, K., & Krause, M. O. (2012). Bridging person-centered outcomes and therapeutic processes for college students with traumatic brain injury. *Perspectives on Neurophysiology and Neurogenic Speech and Language Disorders, 22,* 143–151.

Kennedy, M. R. T., Vaccaro, M., & Hart, T. (2015). Traumatic brain injury: What college disability specialists and educators should know about executive functions. Retrieved from *www.partnership.vcu.edu/TBIresources/downloadables/CollegeStudents_TBI.pdf.*

Kennedy, M. R. T., & Yorkston, K. M. (2000). Accuracy of metamemory after traumatic brain injury: Predictions during verbal learning. *Journal of Speech, Language, and Hearing Research, 43,* 1072–1086.

Kiresuk, T. J., & Sherman, R. (1968). Goal attainment scaling: A general method for evaluating comprehensive community mental health programs. *Community Mental Health Journal, 4,* 443–453.

Kiresuk, T. J., Smith, A., & Cardillo, J. E. (Eds.). (2013). *Goal attainment scaling: Applications, theory, and measurement.* New York: Psychology Press.

Kirkwood, L. (2014). More veterans taking advantage of the Post-911 GI Bill. Retrieved from *www.mcclatchydc.com/2014/03/17/221479/more-veterans-taking-advantage.html.*

Kitsanta, A., Winsler, A., & Huie, F. (2008). Self-regulation and ability predictors of academic success during college: A predictive validity study. *Journal of Advanced Academics, 20*(1), 42–68.

Knollman-Porter, K., Constantinidou, F., & Hutchinson Marron, K. (2014). Speech-language pathology and concussion management in intercollegiate athletics: The Miami University concussion management program. *American Journal of Speech–Language Pathology, 23*(4), 507–519.

Koriat, A., & Bjork, R. A. (2005). Illusions of competence in monitoring one's knowledge during study. *Journal of Experimental Psychology: Learning, Memory, and Cognition, 31*(2), 187–194.

Krasny-Pacini, A., Evans, J., Sohlberg, M. M., & Chevignard, M. (2016). Proposed criteria for appraising goal attainment scales used as outcome measures in rehabilitation research. *Archives of Physical Medicine and Rehabilitation, 97,* 157–170.

Krpan, K. M., Stuss, D. T., & Anderson, N. D. (2011a). Coping behaviour following traumatic brain injury: What makes a planner plan and an avoider avoid? *Brain Injury, 25*(10), 989–996.

Krpan, K. M., Stuss, D. T., & Anderson, N. D. (2011b). Planful versus avoidant coping: Behavior of individuals with moderate-to-severe traumatic brain injury during a psychosocial stress test. *Journal of the International Neuropsychological Society, 17*(2), 248–255.

Kwok, S. T., Wong, W. N., & Lee, K. Y. A. (2014). Effect of resilience on self-perceived stress and experiences on stress symptoms: A surveillance report. *Universal Journal of Public Health, 2*(2), 64–72.

LaBrie, J. W., Cail, J., Pedersen, E. R., & Migliuri, S. (2011). Reducing alcoholic risk in adjudicated male college students: Further validation of a group motivational enhancement intervention. *Journal of Child and Adolescent Substance Abuse, 20*(1), 82–98.

Lange, R. T., Iverson, G. L., & Rose, A. (2010). Post-concussion symptom reporting and the "good-old-days" bias following mild traumatic brain injury. *Archives of Clinical Neuropsychology, 25*(5), 442–450.

Langlois, A., Rutland-Brown, W., & Wald, M. M. (2006). The epidemiology and impact of traumatic brain injury: A brief overview. *Journal of Head Trauma Rehabilitation, 21*(5), 375–378.

Lazarus, R. S., & Folkman, S. (1984). *Stress, appraisal and coping.* New York: Springer.

Lebel, C., & Beaulieu, C. (2011). Longitudinal development of human brain wiring continues from childhood into adulthood. *Journal of Neuroscience, 31*(30), 10937–10947.

Lee, D. H., Oakland, T., Jackson, G., & Glutting, J. (2008). Estimated prevalence of attention-deficit/hyperactivity disorder symptoms among college freshmen: Gender, race, and rater effects. *Journal of Learning Disabilities, 41,* 371–384.

Levine, B., Robertson, I., Clare, L., Carter, G., Wong, J., Wilson, B., et al. (2000). Rehabilitation of executive function: An experimental–clinical validation of goal management training. *Journal of the International Neuropsychological Society, 6,* 299–312.

Lew, L. L., Otis, J. D., Tun, C., Kerns, R. D., Clark, M. E., & Cifu, D. X. (2009). Prevalence of chronic pain, posttraumatic stress disorder, and persistent postconcussive symptoms in OEF/OIF veterans: Polytrauma clinical triad. *Journal of Rehabilitation Research and Development, 46*(6), 697–702.

Lezak, M. D., Howieson, D. B., Bigler, D., & Tranel, D. (2012). *Neuropsychological assessment.* New York: Oxford University Press.

Lichtinger, E., & Kaplan, A. (2015). Employing a case study approach to capture motivation and self-regulation of young students with learning disabilities in authentic educational contexts. *Metacognition and Learning, 10*(1), 119–149.

Litz, B., Stein, N., Delaney, E., Lebowitz, L., Nash, W. P., Silva, C., et al.(2009). Moral injury and moral repair in war veterans: A preliminary model and intervention strategy. *Clinical Psychology Review, 29*(8), 695–706.

Locke, E. A., & Latham, G. P. (2002). New direction in goal-setting theory. *Association for Psychological Science, 1*(5), 265–267.

Lombardi, A., Gerdes, H., & Murray, C. (2011). Validating an assessment of individual actions, postsecondary supports, and social supports of college students with disabilities. *Journal of Student Affairs Research and Practice, 48*(1), 107–126.

Loyens, S. M. M., Magda, J., & Rikers, R. (2008). Self-directed learning in problem-based learning and its relationship with self-regulated learning. *Educational Psychology Review, 20*(4), 411–427.

Lundahl, B. W., Kunz, C., Brownell, C., Tollefson, D., & Burke, B. L. (2010). A meta-analysis of motivational interviewing: Twenty-five years of empirical studies. *Research on Social Work Practice, 20,* 137–160.

Luria, A. R. (1973). *The working brain.* New York: Basic Books.

Luria, A. R. (1980). *Higher cortical functions in man.* New York: Basic Books.

Luxton, D. D., Greenburg, D., Ryan, J., Niven, A., Wheeler, G., & Mysliwiec, V. (2011). Prevalence and impact of short sleep duration in redeployed OIF soldiers. *Sleep, 34*(9), 1189–1195.

MacDonald, S. (2005). *Functional Assessment of Verbal Reasoning and Executive Strategies (FAVRES).* Guelph, ON, Canada: CCD.

MacGregor, A. J., Dougherty, A. L., Tang, J. J., & Galarneau, M. R. (2012). Postconcussive symptom reporting among U.S. combat veterans with mild traumatic brain injury from operation Iraqi freedom. *Journal of Head Trauma Rehabilitation, 28*(1), 59–67.

Madaus, J. W., Miller, W. K., & Vance, M. L. (2009). Veterans with disabilities in postsecondary education. *Journal of Postsecondary Education and Disability, 22*(1), 10–17.

Magill, M., Gaume, J., Apodaca, T., Walthers, J., Mastroleo, N. R., & Borsari, B. (2014). The technical hypothesis of motivational interviewing: A meta-analysis of MI's key causal model. *Journal of Consulting and Clinical Psychology, 82*(6), 973–983.

Malec, J. (2005). The Mayo–Portland Adaptability Inventory. Retrieved March 15, 2016, from *www.tbims.org.combi/mpai.*

Mashima, P., et al. (2017). *Clinician's guide to cognitive rehabilitation in mTBI: Application in military service members and veterans.* Rockville, MD: American Speech-Language-Hearing Association.

Master, C. L., Gioia, G. A., Leddy, J. J., & Grady, M. F. (2012). Importance of 'return-to-learn' in pediatric and adolescent concussion. *Pediatric Annals, 41*(9), 1–6.

Mazzotti, V. L., Kelley, K. R., & Coco, C. M. (2015). Effects of self-directed summary of performance on postsecondary education students' participation in person-centered planning meetings. *Journal of Special Education, 48*(4), 243–255.

McCauley, R. J., & Fey, M. E. (2006). Introduction to treatment of language disorders in children. In R. J. McCauley & M. E. Fey (Eds.), *Treatment of language disorders in children* (pp. 1–17). Baltimore: Brookes.

McClincy, M. P., Lovell, M. R., Pardini, J., Collins, M. W., & Spore, M. K. (2006). Recovery from sports concussion in high school and collegiate athletes. *Brain Injury, 20*(1), 33–39.

McCrea, M., Guskiewicz, K. M., Marshall, S. W., Barr, W., Randolph, C., Cantu, R. C., et al. (2003) Acute effects and recovery time following concussion in collegiate football players: The NCAA concussion study. *Journal of the American Medical Association, 290*(19), 2556–2563.

McCrory, P., Meeuwisse, W., Aubry, M., Cantu, B., Dvorak, J., Echemendia, R., et al. (2013). Consensus statement on concussion in sport: The Fourth International Conference on Concussion in Sport held in Zurich, November 2012. *Journal of Science and Medicine in Sport, 16,* 178–189.

McDonald, S., Togher, L., & Code, C. (Eds.). (2014). *Social and communication disorders following traumatic brain injury* (2nd ed.). New York: Psychology Press.

McFarlane, L. (2012). Motivational interviewing: Practical strategies for speech-language pathologists and audiologists. *Canadian Journal of Speech–Language Pathology and Audiology, 36*(1), 8–16.

McLellan, D. L. (1997). Introduction to rehabilitation. In B. A. Wilson, & D. L. McLellan (Eds.), *Rehabilitation studies handbook.* Cambridge, UK: Cambridge University Press.

Mealings, M., Douglas, J., & Olver, J. (2012). Considering the student perspective in returning to school after TBI: A literature review. *Brain Injury, 26*(10), 1165–1176.

Medley, A. R., & Powell, T. (2010). Motivational interviewing to promote self-awareness and engagement in rehabilitation following acquired brain injury: A conceptual review. *Neuropsychological Rehabilitation, 20*(4), 481–508.

Meulenbroek, P., & Turkstra, L. S. (2016). Job stability in skilled work and communication ability after moderate–severe traumatic brain injury, *Disability and Rehabilitation, 38*(50), 452–461.

Miller, W. R., & Moyers, T. (2006) Eight stages in learning motivational interviewing. *Journal of Teaching the Additions, 5,* 3–17.

Miller, W. R., & Rollnick, S. (2002). *Motivational interviewing: Preparing people for change.* New York: Guilford Press.

Miller, W. R., & Rollnick, S. (2013). *Motivational interviewing: Helping people change* (3rd ed.). New York: Guilford Press.

Mittenburg, W., DiGulio, D. V., Perrin, S., & Bass, A. E. (1992). Symptoms following mild head injury: Expectation as aetiology. *Journal of Neurology, Neurosurgery, and Psychiatry, 55*(3), 200–204.

Miyake, A., Friedman, N. P., Emerson, M. J., Witzki, A. H., & Howerter, A. (2000). The unity and diversity of executive functions and their contributions to complex "frontal lobe" tasks: A latent variable analysis. *Cognitive Psychology, 41*(1), 49–100.

Muraven, M., & Baumeister, R. F. (2000). Self-regulation and depletion of limited resources: Does self-control resemble a muscle? *Psychological Bulletin, 126*(2), 247–259.

Mysliwiec, V., McGraw, L., Pierce, R., Smith, P., Trapp, B., & Roth, B. J. (2013). Sleep disorders and associated medical comorbidities in active duty military personnel. *Sleep, 36*(2), 167–174.

Najavits, L. M., Highley, J., Dolan, S., & Fee, F. A. (2012). Substance use disorder. In J. J. Vasterling, R. A. Bryant, & T. M. Keane (Eds.), *PTSD and mild traumatic brain injury* (pp. 124–145). New York: Guilford Press.

Ness, B. M., Rocke, M. R., Harrist, C. J., & Vroman, K. G. (2014). College and combat trauma: An insider's perspective of the post-secondary education experience shared by service members managing neurobehavioral symptoms. *NeuroRehabilitation, 35*(1), 147–158.

Ness, B. M. & Vroman, K. (2014). Preliminary examination of the impact of traumatic brain injury and posttraumatic stress disorder on self-regulated learning and academic achievement among military service members enrolled in postsecondary education. *Journal of Head Trauma Rehabilitation, 29*(1), 33–43.

O'Brien, K., Schellinger, S., & Kennedy, M. R. T. (2017). Strategy outcomes from coaching college students with traumatic brain injury.

O'Neil-Pirozzi, T., Kennedy, M. R. T., & Sohlberg, M. M. (2016). Evidence-based practice for the use of internal strategies as a memory compensation technique after brain injury: A systematic review. *Journal of Head Trauma Rehabilitation, 31*(4), E1–E11.

Oaten, M., & Cheng, K. (2005). Academic examination stress impairs self–control. *Journal of Social and Clinical Psychology, 24*(2), 254–279.

Ownsworth, T., McFarland, K. & Young, R. M. (2000). Development and standardization of the self-regulation skills interview (SRSI): A new clinical assessment tool for acquired brain injury. *The Clinical Neuropsychologist, 14*(1), 76–92.

Park, C. L., Edmundson, D., & Lee, J. (2011). Development of self-regulation abilities as predictors of psychological adjustment across the first year of college. *Journal of Adult Development, 19*(1), 40–49.

Parker, D. R., & Boutelle, K. (2009). Executive function coaching for college students with learning disabilities and ADHD: A new approach for fostering self-determination. *Learning Disabilities Research and Practice, 24*(4), 204–215.

Parker, D. R., Field, S., Hoffman, S. F., Sawilowsky, S., & Rolands, L. (2011). Self-control in postsecondary settings: Students' perceptions of ADHD college coaching. *Journal of Attention Disorders, 17*(3), 215–232.

Pham, L. B., & Taylor, S. E. (1999). From thought to action: Effects of process- versus outcome-based mental simulations on performance. *Personality and Social Psychology Bulletin, 25*, 250–260.

Pintrich, P. R., & DeGroot, E. V. (1990). Motivational and self-regulated learning components of classroom academic performance. *Journal of Education Psychology, 82*(1), 33–40.

Polley, M., Frank, D., & Smith, M. (2012). National Veteran Sleep Survey: Results and findings. Retrieved from *http://myvetadvisor.com/wp-content/uploads/2013/07/Vetadvisor_sleepreport-1.pdf.*

Polusny, M. A., Kehle, S. M., Nelson, N. W., Erbes, C. R., Arbisi, P. A., & Thuras, P. (2011). Longitudinal effects of mild TBI and PTSD comorbidity on post-deployment outcomes in national guard soldiers deployed to Iraq. *Archives of General Psychiatry, 68*(1), 79–89.

Ponsford, J., Bayley, M., Wiseman-Hakes, C., Togher, L., Velikonja, D., McIntyre, A., et al. (2014). INCOG Recommendations for management of cognition following traumatic brain injury: Part II. Attention and information processing speed. *Journal of Head Trauma Rehabilitation, 29*(4), 321–337.

Prochaska, J. O., DiClemente, C. C., & Norcross, J. C. (1992). In search of how people change. *American Psychologist, 47*(9), 1102–1114.

Quinn, P. O., Ratey, N., & Maitland, T. L. (2000). *Coaching college students with AD/HD: Issues and answers.* Spring Silver, MD: Advantage Books.

Rabiner, D. L., Anastopoulos, A. D., Costello, J., Hoyle, R. H., & Swartzwelder, H. S. (2008). Adjustment to college in students with ADHD. *Journal of Attention Disorders, 11,* 689–699.

Randolph, C. (2012). *The Repeatable Battery for the Assessment of Neuropsychological Status.* San Antonio, TX: Pearson Education.

Raue, K., & Lewis, L. (2011). *Students with disabilities at degree-granting postsecondary institutions.* (NCES 2011-018). Washington, DC: U.S. Government Printing Office.

Reaser, A., Prevatt, F., Petscher, Y., & Proctor, B. (2007). The learning and study strategies of college students with ADHD. *Psychology in the Schools, 44*(6), 627–638.

Ribeiro, J. D., Pease, J. L., Gutierrez, P. M., Silva, C., Bernert, R. A., Rudd, M. D., et al. (2012). Sleep problems outperform depression and hopelessness as cross-sectional and longitudinal predictors of suicidal ideation and behavior in young adults in the military. *Journal of Affective Disorders, 136*(3), 743–750.

Richardson, M., Abraham, C., & Bond, R. (2012). Psychological correlates of university students' academic performance: A systematic review and meta-analysis. *Psychological Bulletin, 138*(2), 353–387.

Robertson, I. H., Ward, T., Ridgeway, V., & Nimmo-Smith, I. (1994). *Test of Everyday Attention.* Suffolk, UK: Thames Valley Test Company.

Rosengren, D. B. (2009). *Building motivational interviewing skills: A practitioner workbook.* New York: Guilford Press.

Roth, R. M., Lance, C. E., Isquith, P. K., Fischer, A. S., & Giancola, P. R. (2013). Confirmatory factor analysis of the behavior rating inventory of executive function-adult version in healthy adults and application to attention-deficit/hyperactivity disorder. *Clinical Neuropsychology, 28*(5), 425–434.

Roth, R. S., & Spencer, R. J. (2013). Iatrogenic risk in the management of mild traumatic brain injury among combat veterans: A case illustration and commentary. *International Journal of Physical Medicine and Rehabilitation, 1*(1), 1–7.

Rubak, S., Sandbaek, A., Lauritzen, T., & Christensen, B. (2005). Motivational interviewing: A systematic review and analysis. *British Journal of General Practice, 55,* 305–312.

Ruff, R. M., Light, R. H., Parker, S. B., & Levin, H. S. (1996), Benton Controlled Oral Word Association Test: Reliability and updated norms. *Archives of Clinical Neuropsychology, 11*(4), 329–338.

Rumann, C. B., & Hamrick, F. A. (2010). Student veterans in transition: Re-enrolling after warzone deployment. *Journal of Higher Education, 81*(4), 431–458.

Ryan, A. M., & Pintrich, P. R. (1997). Should I ask for help?: The role of motivation and attitudes in adolescents' help seeking in math class. *Journal of Educational Psychology, 89,* 329–341.

Salthouse, T. A., Atkinson, T. M., & Berish, D. E. (2003). Executive functioning as a potential mediator of age-related cognitive decline in normal adults. *Journal of Experimental Psychology, 132*(4), 566–594.

Sarason, I. G., Sarason, B. R., Shearin, E. N., & Pierce, G. R. (1987). A brief measure of social support: Practical and theoretical implications. *Journal of Social and Personal Relationships, 4*, 497–510.

Schefft, B. K., Dulay, M. F., & Fargo, J. D. (2008). The use of a self-generation memory encoding strategy to improve verbal memory and learning in patients with traumatic brain injury. *Application of Neuropsychology, 15*(1), 61–68.

Schell, T. L., & Marshall, G. N. (2008). *Survey of individuals previously deployed for OEF/OIF.* Santa Monica, CA: RAND.

Schmidt, J., Lannin, N., Fleming, J., & Ownsworth, T. (2011). Feedback interventions for impaired self-awareness following brain injury: A systematic review. *Journal of Rehabilitation Medicine, 43*(8), 673–680.

Schunk, D. H. (1991). Self-efficacy and academic motivation. *Educational Psychologist, 26*(3–4), 207–231.

Scott, S. (2002). The dynamic process of providing accommodations. In L. C. Brinckerhoff, J. M. McGuire, & S. F. Shaw, *Postsecondary education and transition for students with learning disabilities* (2nd ed., pp. 295–332). Austin, TX: PRO-ED.

Shackelford, A. L. (2009). Documenting the needs of student veterans with disabilities: Intersection roadblocks, solutions, and legal realities. *Journal of Postsecondary Education, 22*(1), 36–42.

Shaw-Zirt, B., Popali-Lehane, L., Chaplin, W., & Bergman, A. (2005). Adjustment, social skills, and self-esteem in college students with symptoms of ADHD. *Journal of Attention Disorders, 8*, 109–120.

Shinseki, E. K. (2013, April 16). Remarks by Secretary Eric K. Shinseki. Senator Sherrod Brown's Ohio College Presidents Conference. Retrieved from *www.va.gov/opa/speeches/2013/04_16_2013.asp.*

Shively, S. B., & Perl, D. P. (2012). Traumatic brain injury, shell shock, and posttraumatic stress disorder in the military: Past, present, and future. *Journal of Head Trauma Rehabilitation, 27*(3), 234–239.

Sitzman, T., & Ely, K. (2011). A meta-analysis of self-regulated learning in work-related and educational attainment: What we know and where we need to go. *Psychological Bulletin, 137*(3), 421–442.

Smee, D., Buenrostro, S., Garrick, T., Sreenivasan, S., & Weinberger, L. E. (2013). Combat to college: Cognitive fatigue as a challenge in Iraq and Afghanistan war veterans with traumatic brain injury: Pilot study survey results. *Journal of Applied Rehabilitation Counseling, 44*(4), 25–33.

Smith, B. W., Dalen, J., Wiggins, K., Tooley, E., Christopher, P., & Bernard, J. (2008). The brief resilience scale: Assessing the ability to bounce back. *International Journal of Behavioral Medicine, 15*(3), 194–200.

Sohlberg, M. M., Ehlardt, L., & Kennedy, M. (2005). Instructional techniques in cognitive rehabilitation: A preliminary report. *Seminars in Speech and Language, 26*(4), 268–279.

Sohlberg, M. M., & Tursktra, L. (2011). *Optimizing cognitive rehabilitation.* New York: Guilford Press.

Solberg, V. S., O'Brien, K., Villareal, P., Kennel, R., & Davis, B. (1993). Self-efficacy and Hispanic college students: Validation of the college self-efficacy instrument. *Hispanic Journal of Behavioral Sciences, 15*(1), 80–95.

Squire, L. R. (1992). Declarative and nondeclarative memory: Multiple brain systems supporting learning and memory. *Journal of Cognitive Neuroscience, 4*(3), 232–243.

Steptoe, A., Wardle, J., Pollard, T. M., Canaan, L., & Davies, G. J. (1996). Stress, social support and health-related behavior: A study of smoking, alcohol consumption and physical exercise. *Journal of Psychosomatic Research, 41*(2), 171–180.

Stuss, D., & Benson, D. F. (1986). *The frontal lobes.* New York: Raven Press.

Swanson, H. L. (1999). Instructional components that predict treatment outcomes for students with learning disabilities: Support for the combined strategy and direct instruction model. *Learning Disabilities Research and Practice, 14,* 129–140.

Swanson, H. L., & Deshler, D. (2003). Instructing adolescents with learning disabilities: Converting a meta-analysis to practice, *Journal of Learning Disabilities, 36*(2), 124–135.

Swanson, H. L., & Hoskyn, M. (1998). Experimental intervention research on students with learning disabilities: A meta-analysis of treatment outcomes. *Review of Educational Research, 68*(3), 277–321.

Swartz, S. L., Prevatt, F., & Proctor, B. E. (2005). A coaching intervention for college students with attention deficit/hyperactivity disorder. *Psychology in the Schools, 42*(6), 647–656.

Tanelian, T., & Jaycox, L. H. (2008). *Invisible wounds of war: Psychological and cognitive injuries, their consequences, and services to assist recovery.* Santa Monica, CA: RAND.

Tate, R., Kennedy, M. R. T., Bayley, M., Bragge, P., Douglas, J., Kita, M., et al. (2014). INCOG recommendations for management of cognition following traumatic brain injury: Part VI. Executive function and self-awareness. *Journal of Head Trauma Rehabilitation, 29*(4), 338–352.

Taylor, S. E. (2011). Envisioning the future and self-regulation. In M. Bar (Ed.), *Predictions in the brain: Using our past to generate a future* (pp. 134–143). New York: Oxford University Press.

Terrio, H., Brenner, L. A., Ivins, B. J., Cho, J. M., Helmick, K., Schwab, K., et al. (2009). Traumatic brain injury screening: Preliminary findings in a US Army Brigade Combat Team. *Journal of Head Trauma Rehabilitation, 24*(1), 14–23.

Tick, E. (2005). *War and the soul.* Wheaton, IL: Quest Books.

Toglia, J., Johnston, M. V., Goverover, Y., & Dain, B. (2010). A multicontext approach to promoting transfer of strategy use and self-regulation after brain injury: An exploratory study. *Brain Injury, 24*(4), 664–677.

Troxel, W. M., Shih, R. A., Pedersen, E., Geyer, L., Fisher, M. P., Griffin, B. A., et al. (2015). *Sleep in the military: Promoting healthy sleep among U.S. service members.* Santa Monica, CA: RAND.

Turkstra, L. S., Politis, A. M., & Forsyth, R. (2015). Cognitive-communication disorders in children with traumatic brain injury. *Developmental Medicine and Child Neurology, 57*(3), 217–222.

Turkstra, L. S., Ylvisaker, M., Coelho, C., Kennedy, M. R. T., Sohlberg, M. M., & Avery, J. (2005). Practice guidelines for standardized assessment for persons with traumatic brain injury. *Journal of Medical Speech–Language Pathology, 13*(2), 9–38.

U.S. Department of Veterans Affairs. (2015, June 3). Polytrauma/TBI system of care. Retrieved from *www.polytrauma.va.gov/definitions.asp.*

Van Dongen, H. P. A., Maislin, G., Mullington, J. M., & Dinges, D. F. (2003). The cumulative cost of additional wakefulness: Dose–response effects on neurobehavioral functions and sleep physiology from chronic sleep restriction and total sleep deprivation. *Sleep, 26*(6), 117–126.

Vance, M. L., & Miller, W. K. (2009). Serving wounded warriors: Current practices in post-secondary education. *Journal of Postsecondary Education, 22*(1), 18–35.

Vasterling, J. J., & Brailey, K. (2005). Neuropsychological findings in adults with PTSD. In J. J. Vasterling & C. R. Brewin (Eds.), *Neuropsychology of PTSD. Biological, cognitive, and clinical perspectives* (pp. 178–207). New York: Guilford Press.

Vasterling, J. J., Brailey, K., Constans, J. I., & Sutker, P. B. (1998). Attention and memory dysfunction in posttraumatic stress disorder. *Neuropsychology, 12*(1), 125–133.

Vasterling, J. J., Bryant, R. A., & Keane, T. M. (2012). *PTSD and mild traumatic brain injury.* New York: Guilford Press.

Vasterling, J. J., Proctor, S. P., Amoroso, P., Kane, R., Heeren, T., & White, R. F. (2006). Neuropsychological outcomes of army personnel following deployment to the Iraq war. *Journal of the American Medical Association, 296*(5), 519–529.

Vasterling, J. J., Verfaellie, M., & Sullivan, K. D. (2009). Mild traumatic brain injury and posttraumatic stress disorder in returning veterans: Perspectives from cognitive neuroscience. *Clinical Psychology Review, 29*(8), 674–684.

Velikonja, D., Tate, R., Ponsford, K., McIntyre, A., Janzen, S., & Bayley, M. (2014). INCOG recommendations for management of cognition following traumatic brain injury: Part V. Memory. *Journal of Head Trauma Rehabilitation, 29*(4), 369–286.

Von Korff, M., Dworkin, S. F., Le Resche, L., & Kruger, A. (1988). An epidemiologic comparison of pain complaints. *Pain, 32*(2), 173–183.

Walker, Q. D. (2010). An investigation of the relationship between career maturity, career decision self-efficacy, and self-advocacy of college students with and without disabilities. *Dissertation Abstracts International, Section A, 71*, 2372.

Wallace, B. A., Winsler, A., & NeSmith, P. (1999, April 19–23). *Factors associated with success for college students with ADHD: Are standard accommodations helping?* Paper presented at the annual meeting of the American Educational Research Association, Montreal, Quebec, Canada.

Wambaugh, J. L. (2007). The evidence-based practice and practice-based evidence nexus. *Perspectives on Neurophysiology and Neurogenic Speech and Language Disorders, 17*(1), 732–742.

Warden, D. (2006). Military TBI during the Iraq and Afghanistan wars. *Journal of Head Trauma Rehabilitation, 21*(5), 398–402.

Watson Institute for International and Public Affairs, Brown University. (n.d.). U.S. veterans and military families. Retrieved from *http://watson.brown.edu/costsofwar/costs/human/veterans.*

Wechsler, D. (2001). *Wechsler Test of Adult Reading.* San Antonio, TX: Pearson Education.

Wechsler, D. (2009). *Wechsler Adult Memory Scale–IV.* San Antonio, TX: Pearson Education.

Wehman, P. (2010). *Essentials of transition planning.* Baltimore: Brookes.

Weinstein, C. E., & Palmer, D. R. (2002) *LASSI: Learning and Study Strategies Inventory, 2nd edition.* Clearwater, FL: H & H.

West, R., & Lennox, S. (1992). Function of cigarette smoking in relation to examinations. *Psychopharmacology, 108*(4), 456–459.

Willcutt, E. G., Doyle, A. E., Nigg, J. T., Faraone, S. V., & Pennington, B. F. (2005). Validity of the executive function theory of attention-deficit/hyperactivity disorder: A meta-analytic review. *Biological Psychiatry, 57*(11), 1336–1346.

Willmott, C., Ponsford J., Downing M., & Carty, M. (2014). Frequency and quality of return to study following traumatic brain injury. *Journal of Head Trauma Rehabilitation, 29,* 248–256.

Wilson, B. (2003). Goal planning rather than neuropsychological tests should be used to structure and evaluate cognitive rehabilitation. *Brain Impairment, 4*(1), 25–30.

Winkens, I., Van Heugten, C., Wade, D., & Fasotti, L. (2009). Training patients in time pressure management: A cognitive strategy for mental slowness. *Clinical Rehabilitation, 23,* 79–90.

Wood, R. L. (2007). Post concussional syndrome: All in the mind's eye! *Journal of Neurology, Neurosurgery and Psychiatry, 78*(6), 552.

Wyble, B., Sharma, D., & Bowman, H. (2008). Strategic regulation of cognitive control by emotional salience: A neural network model. *Cognition and Emotion, 22*(6), 1019–1051.

Wyman P. A., Cowen, E. L., Work, W. C., & Parker, G. R. (1991). Developmental and family milieu correlates of resilience in urban children who have experienced major life stress. *American Journal of Community Psychology, 19,* 405–426.

Ylvisaker, M. (1998). *Everyday routines in traumatic brain injury rehabilitation.* Rockville, MD: American Speech–Language–Hearing Association.

Ylvisaker, M. (2006). Self-coaching: A context-sensitive, person-centered approach to social communication after traumatic brain injury. *Brain Impairment, 7*(3), 246–258.

Ylvisaker, M., & Feeney, T. (1998). *Collaborative brain injury intervention.* San Diego, CA: Singular.

Ylvisaker, M., & Feeney, T. (2009). Executive functions, self-regulation and learned optimism in pediatric rehabilitation: A review and suggestions for intervention. *Pediatric Rehabilitation, 6*(1), 57–60.

Ylvisaker, M., Turkstra, L., Coelho, C., Kennedy, M. R. T., Sohlberg, M. M., & Yorkston, K. M. (2007). Behavioral interventions for individuals with behavior disorders after traumatic brain injury: A systematic review. *Brain Injury, 21*(8), 769–805.

Zajacova, A., Lynch, S. M., & Espenshade, T. J. (2005). Self-efficacy, stress, and academic success in college. *Research in Higher Education, 46*(6), 677–706.

Zimmerman, B. J., & Martinez-Pons, M. (1986). Development of a structured interview for assessing student use of self-regulated learning strategies. *American Educational Research Journal, 23*(4), 614–628.

Zwart, L. M., & Kallemeyn, L. M. (2001). Peer-based coaching for college students with ADHD and learning disabilities. *Journal of Postsecondary Education and Disability, 15*(1), 1–15.

Index

Page numbers that are italicized denote a figure or a table.

ABI. *See* Acquired brain injury
Academic counseling, 49
Academic self-efficacy, 51–52
Academic Statements from the CCS-OD, CSS-BI, and the CSS-C, with Importance Ratings and Follow-Up Questions (Form 5.7), 103, 113, 143–148
Academic stress, 20
Academic success, veterans and, 51–52
Accommodations
  coaching self-advocacy regarding, 203, 205, *206*
  types available and concerns regarding, 196–198
Acquired brain injury (ABI)
  college students with, executive function problems and, 28–32
  definition and categories of, 28
  motivational interviewing and, 64–65
  prevalence, 28–29
  student benefits associated with dynamic coaching, 79–80
Action phase/stage
  self-regulation process, *74*, 75–77
  stages of change coaching model, 59, *61*
Action-Planning Form (Form 4.6), 77, 88–89, *165–166*, 201, *202*, *203*
Action plans, 76
ADHD. *See* Attention-deficit/hyperactivity disorder
Adjustment phase, 77–78
Affirming, in motivational interviewing, 64, *65*
Afghanistan war veterans. *See* Military service members and veterans
After-action reviews, 52
Alertness, *9*
American Speech–Language–Hearing Association, 70
Americans with Disabilities Act (ADA), 195

Americans with Disabilities Act Amendment Act of 2008, 47, 195
Anxiety, 50–51
Any.Do (time-management app), *178*
Apple time-management apps, 177, *178*
Apps. *See* Mobile applications
ASD. *See* Autism spectrum disorder
Attention/Attention control, *9*, *13*
Attention deficit disorder (ADD), 26
Attention-deficit/hyperactivity disorder (ADHD)
  college students with
    benefits associated with dynamic coaching, 79
    coaching models, 59, 61–62
    enrollment at postsecondary institutions, 23–24
    example of information gathering with, 96
  executive function problems and, 26–27
  motivational interviewing and, 64
Autism spectrum disorder (ASD)
  college students with, enrollment at postsecondary institutions, 23–24
  executive function problems and, 27–28
Autobiographical beliefs, 16
Automatic behaviors, 14–15
Autonomic/emotional processes, *9–10*
Avoidant coping styles, 66

Battle fatigue, 39
Battlemind, 44–45
Behavioral flexibility, *13*
Behavioral regulation, 12
Behavior Rating Inventory of Executive Function (BRIEF), 12
Behavior Rating Inventory of Executive Function—Adult Version (BRIEF-A), 31, *99*, 101

"Better Google Tasks" (time-management app), *178*
Blast exposure, 37–39
Brief Resilience Scale (BRS), *101*, 102, 114

Chronic pain, 39, 40
Coaching models, for students with executive function
    problems, 58–62
Coaching sessions, weekly, value of, 69–70, 118
Cognitive flexibility, *13*
Cognitive/intellectual impairment
    college students with, enrollment at postsecondary
        institutions, 23–24
    executive function problems and, 27–28
Cognitive processes
    challenges with military service members and
        veterans, 51–52
    executive functions and, 8–11
Cognitive rehabilitation therapy, 215
Cognitive self-regulation
    functions of and manifestations of impairment in, *13*
    impact of emotional self-regulation on, 18–19
Collaborative coaching model, 59
Collaborative goal setting, 109
Collaborative planning
    development of a coaching plan, 114–118
    documenting outcomes, 112–114
    identifying multiple outcomes and multiple goals,
        108–112
    interpreting abilities and disabilities, 107
    overview, 68, 93, 107
Collaborative relationship
    building through dynamic coaching, 63–66
    importance in the self-regulation process, 75
College faculty and administrative staff, 53
College life, difficulties navigating for military service
    members and veterans, 49–50
College Self-Efficacy Inventory (CSEI), *99*, 101, 114
College students
    basic roles and responsibilities of, *194*
    See also Executive function problems, college students
        with; Military service members and veterans
College Students with Disabilities Campus Climate
    (CSDCC), *99*, 113
College Survey for Students with Brain Injury (CSS-BI;
    Form 5.5), *99*, 102, 103, 105, 113, 130–135, 147
College Survey for Students with Concussion (CSS-C;
    Form 5.6), 102, 103, 105, 113, 136–142, 148–149
College Survey for Students with Concussion and Other
    Injuries (CSS-CO), *99*, 102, 103
College Survey for Students with Other Disabilities
    (CSS-OD; Form 5.4), *99*, 102, 103, 105, 113,
    125–130, 145–146
College Well-Being Scale (CWBS), 79, *99*
Combat deployment
    alterations in neural functioning and, 39
    effects on college performance of veterans, 48
Combat fatigue, 39
Communication strategies, for self-advocacy, *207*
Concussion (mild traumatic brain injury)
    defined, 28
    management when returning to college, 31–32

in military service members and veterans
    from blast exposure, 37–39
    misattribution of symptoms and iatrogenesis, 42–43
    sleep disorders and, 40
    prevalence, 28–29
    symptoms and executive function problems, 30–31
    what disability service specialists should know about,
        33–36
Contemplation stage, 59, *60*
Context, self-coaching and, 59
Context-based learning, 70–72
Controlled Word Association Test (COWAT), *99*
Coping styles, 66
CSS surveys, 102–107

Daily Goals ("habit tracker" app), 185
Demographic, Academic, Medical, and Social History
    Form (Form 5.3), 95, 121–124
Depression, 41
Developmental disabilities, college students with
    ADHD, 25, 26–27
    autism spectrum disorder and intellectual disability,
        27–28
    characterization of experiences in college, 24–25
    enrollment at postsecondary institutions, 23–24
    learning disabilities, 25–26, 27
Didactic instruction, dynamic coaching approach
    compared to, *78*
Direct instruction of self-regulation, 73
Disability services
    basic roles and responsibilities of, *194*
    information gathering about students' use of, 105–107
    need for by military service members and veterans in
        college, 46–48
    students with personal barriers to self-advocacy and,
        193–195
Discrimination, student protections against, 195–196
Distal goals
    defined, 108
    in the development of a coaching plan, 114, 115, *116*
    documenting outcomes, 113–114
Dual disabilities
    acquired brain injury and executive function
        problems, 28–32
    college students with, enrollment at postsecondary
        institutions, 23–25
    defined, 11
    developmental disabilities and executive function
        problems, 25–28
Dynamic coaches
    billing for services, 215
    integrating the dynamic coaching approach into one's
        practice, 214–216
    requirements for, 58
    what good coaches do and do not do, *68*
Dynamic coaching approach
    additional resources, 82
    coaching self-advocacy. *See* Self-advocacy
    coaching self-learning. *See* Self-learning coaching
    coaching self-management. *See* Self-management
        coaching

collaborative planning. *See* Collaborative planning
collaborative relationship building, 63–66
compared to didactic instruction, 78
context-based learning and, 70–72
fostering self-coaching, 212–214
information gathering. *See* Information gathering
instructing self-regulation, 72–78
integrating into one's practice, 214–216
introduction to and overview of, 57–58, 62
origins and applicability of, 1–3
requirements for dynamic coaches, 58
structuring to model and facilitate self-regulation, 66–70
student benefits associated with, 79–82

Elaborative encoding strategy, *171*
Emotional self-regulation
    functions of and manifestations of impairment in, *13*
    impact on cognitive self-regulation, 18–19
Environmental structuring strategies, 172–173
Erikson, Erik, 42
Evernote (time-management app), *178*
Evidence-based strategies, in the self-regulation process, 75
Executive function problems
    affecting military service members and veterans. *See* Military service members and veterans
    barriers to self-advocacy, 191–192
    college students with
        acquired brain injury and, 28–32
        characterization of experiences in college, 24–25
        developmental disabilities and, 25–28
        enrollment at postsecondary institutions, 22–24
        models for coaching, 58–62
        overview, 22
    information gathering about. *See* Information gathering
    self-regulation and, 20–21
Executive functions
    automatic behaviors and, 14–15
    dual disabilities, 11
    frameworks for understanding functions and impairments of, 8–12, *13*
    integrative nature of, 11
    reasons for different lists of, 12, 14
    self-regulation and, 7, 15, 19, 21
    supplemental tests for information gathering, 97–98

Feedback, self-regulation and, 17
Finish (time-management app), *178*
Flashcards, 171
Frontal lobe strokes, 32
Functional Assessment of Verbal Reasoning and Executive Strategies (FAVRES), 98, *100*

Generation effect, 71–72
Getting Started Checklist for Coaches (Form 5.1), 94, 119
Getting Started Checklist for Students (Form 5.2), 94–95, 120
Goal attainment scaling (GAS), 110, 164, 208–209

Goal setting
    in the development of a coaching plan, 114–118
    functions of and manifestations of impairment in, *13*
    in self-learning, 162–166
    in self-management, 166–170
Goals
    in the development of a coaching plan, 114–118
    identifying, 108–112
    self-identifying in self-learning, 162–163
    in the self-regulation process, 74–75
    See also Distal goals; Performance goals; Proximal goals; Self-regulation goals
Goals on Track ("habit tracker" app), 185
Goals–Strategies–Act–Adjust (GSAA)
    adjustment phase in self-learning and self-management, 186–188
    coaching self-advocacy, 201–210
    goal setting in self-learning, 162–166, *164*
    goal setting in self-management, 166–170
    instructing self-regulation through dynamic coaching, 73–78
    strategizing for self-learning, 170–174
    strategizing for self-management, 174–182
    tracking strategies and performance in self-learning and self-management, 184–186
Google Keep (time-management app), *178*
Google Tasks (time-management app), *178*
Google time-management apps, 177, *178*
Grade point averages (GPAs), 19
Grades and test scores, 113
GSAA. *See* Goals–Strategies–Act–Adjust

HabitBull ("habit tracker" app), 185
Habit List ("habit tracker" app), 185
"Habit Trackers" apps, 185
Headaches, 40
Help-seeking behaviors, self-advocacy and, 192–193
Hyperarousal/Hypervigilance, 50–51

Iatrogenesis, 43
Immediate goals. *See* Proximal goals
Impulse control, *13*
Independence, coaching toward, 212–214
Independence and follow-up phase, *66*, 69
Information gathering
    flowchart of components and steps in, *94*
    key questions in, 93–96
    overview, 92–93
    supplemental tests, 96–98
    surveys, questionnaires, and interviews, 98–107
Information gathering and evaluating phase, *66*, 68
Inhibition, 11, *13*
Initiation, *13*
Interpreting Abilities and Disabilities (Form 5.8), 107, 149–150
Interpreting and planning phase, *66*, 68
Interviews
    information gathering with, 103–10
    with military service members and veterans, 45–46
Iraq war veterans. *See* Military service members and veterans

Language processes, *10*
Learning and studying
    context-based, 70–72
    learning effects, 161
    metacognitive aspects of, 161–162
    strategizing for, 170–174
    in the support and instruction phase of coaching, 68
    See also Self-learning coaching
Learning and Study Strategies Inventory—2nd Edition
        (LASSI), 27, 79, *100*, 101
Learning disabilities (LD)
    college students with, enrollment at postsecondary
        institutions, 23–24
    college students with executive function problems,
        25–26, 27
    student benefits associated with dynamic coaching,
        79
Learning effects, 161
Left-hemisphere frontal lobe stroke, 32
Listastic (time-management app), *179*
List of Goals by Immediacy, Ranging from Weeks to
        Years (Form 5.10), 117, 156
Long-range goals. *See* Distal goals
Long-term assignments, strategizing for self-
        management, 180–182

Maintenance stage, *61*
Major depressive disorder (MDD), 41
Major depressive episodes (MDE), 41
Mapping Proximal and Distal Goals onto a Plan by
        Immediacy of Need (Form 5.11), 117, 157, 174
Mayo–Portland Adaptability Inventory (MPAI-IV), *100*,
        101
Medical records, 46
Memory impairments
    goal setting in self-learning, 163–164, *165–166*
    manifestations, *9*, *13*
Mental set shifting, 11
Metacognition
    executive functions and, 12
    self-regulation and, 15
Metacognitive beliefs
    self-regulation and, 17–18
    sense of self, 16
Metacognitive strategy instruction, 73
Metamemory, 15
Mild traumatic brain injury. *See* Concussion
Military culture
    overview and relationship to college experiences,
        43–44
    social relationships and, 50
    understanding to provide competent professional
        services, 45–46
Military rank and occupation, 45–46
Military service members and veterans
    blast and traumatic brain injury, 37–39
    chronic pain, 40
    combat deployment and alterations in neural
        functioning, 39
    depression and moral injury, 41–42
    educational context

academic counseling and navigating college life,
        49–50
    additional resources, 53–54
    cognitive challenges, 51–52
    hyperarousal and anxiety, 50–51
    military culture and battle mind, 43–46
    military culture and social relationships, 50
    need for supports, 46–52
    summary of recommendations for, 52–53
    misattribution of symptoms and iatrogenesis, 42–43
    posttraumatic stress disorder, 39–40
    sleep disorders, 40–41
    substance use, 42
Military-to-school transition, 49–50
Misdiagnosis, 42–43
Mobile applications (apps)
    for time management, 177–179
    for tracking strategy use in self-learning and self-
        management, 185
Momentum ("habit tracker" app), 185
Moral injury, 42
Motivational interviewing (MI), 57, 63–66
Motivational Studying and Learning Questionnaire
        (MSLQ), *100*, 101
Motor processes, *10*

Nelson–Denny Reading Test, *100*
Neuroasthenia, 39
Nontraumatic brain injuries, 32
Note-taking strategies, *171*, *172*, *173*, 186–187

OARS (Open questions, Affirming, Reflecting, and
        Summarizing), 64, *65*
Open questions, 64, *65*
Operation Enduring Freedom (OEF) veterans. *See*
        Military service members and veterans
Operation Iraqi Freedom (OIF) veterans. *See* Military
        service members and veterans
Operation New Dawn (OND) veterans. *See* Military
        service members and veterans
Outcomes
    documenting, 112–114
    identifying and framing as goals, 108–112

Partial sleep deprivation, 41
PBE. *See* Practiced-based evidence
PCS. *See* Post-concussive syndrome
Peers, coaching self-advocacy with, 205, 207–209
PEI. *See* Planning, Implementation, and Evaluation
Performance goals
    overview and description of, 110–112
    pairing with self-regulation goals in time
        management, 168–170
    for self-advocacy, 201
    in self-learning, 162–163
Persistence, 80–82
Plan–Do–Review (Form 6.1), 179–180, 189
Planners, traditional, 179
Planning, Implementation, and Evaluation (PIE), 66–70
Planning/preparation stage, 59, *60*
Pocket List (time-management app), *178*

Polytrauma clinical triad, 39
Portfolios, 213
Post-9/11 GI Bill, 46–48
Post-concussive syndrome (PCS), 33–36
Posttraumatic stress disorder (PTSD)
    description of, 39–40
    effects on college performance, 48
    sleep disorders and, 40
    trimorbid disorder and, 42
Practiced-based evidence (PBE), 72
Precontemplation stage, 60
Prediction–performance contrast, 179–180
Preparation/planning stage, 59, 60
Preview–Question–Review–Study–Test (PQRST), 171
Problem-based learning, 61–62
Problem-focused students, 66
Problem identification, 13
Problem solving, 59
Prochaska's stages of change. See Stages of change
        coaching model
Procrastination, 182–183
Productive ("habit tracker" app), 185
Proximal goals
    defined, 108
    in the development of a coaching plan, 114, 115, 116,
        117–118
    outcomes, 114
    pairing self-regulation goals with, 117–118
PTSD. See Posttraumatic stress disorder

Questionnaires, 98–102
Questions, in motivational interviewing, 64, 65

Rating scales, in goal attainment scaling, 110
Reading comprehension strategies, 173
Recall, 71–72
Reciprocal adjusting, 59
Reflecting, in motivational interviewing, 64, 65
Rehabilitation Act (1973), 195
Relationship building, collaborative, 63–66
Remember the Milk (time-management app), 178
Repeatable Battery for Assessment of
        Neuropsychological Status (RBANS), 98, 100
Repetition strategy, 182, 183–184
Reporting, on strategy use, 76–77
Resiliency, 80–82
Retrieval techniques, 171
Right-hemisphere frontal lobe stroke, 32

Self-advocacy
    accommodations, 196–198
    additional resources, 210
    coaching
        GSAA approach, 201–210
        overview of, 190–191
        team approach, 199–201
    communication strategies for college students with
        executive function problems, 207
    definition of, 190
    importance and value to college students, 190, 191
    personal barriers to, 191–195

student protection against discrimination, 195–196
    in the support and instruction phase of coaching, 68
Self-assessment, 15–16
Self-awareness
    cognition and, 8
    metacognitive beliefs and, 16
    self-regulation and, 17–18
Self-coaching, 59, 212–214
Self-control, self-regulation and, 15–16, 17
Self-efficacy (self-determination)
    concept of, 18
    context-based learning and, 71
    GPAs and, 19
Self-evaluations, 52, 73–75
Self-generation, 71–72
Self-learning coaching
    additional resources, 188
    goal setting, 162–166
    Goals–Strategies–Act–Adjust framework, 159
    learning effects, 161
    managing ineffective strategies, 182–184
    metacognitive aspects of learning and, 161–162
    overview, 159–160
    replacing students' ineffective strategies, 160–161
    strategizing for, 170–174
    strategy usefulness and next steps, 186–188
    tracking strategies and performance, 184–186
Self-management coaching
    additional resources, 188
    goal setting, 166–170
    Goals–Strategies–Act–Adjust framework, 159
    managing ineffective strategies, 182–184
    overview, 159–160
    replacing students' ineffective strategies, 160–161
    strategizing for, 174–182
    strategy usefulness and next steps, 186–188
    tracking strategies and performance, 184–186
Self-monitoring, self-regulation and, 15–16, 17
Self-Reflection: End (Form 4.3), 69, 85, 213
Self-Reflection: Start (Form 4.2), 69, 84, 213
Self-reflections
    forms for facilitating, 69
    fostering self-coaching and, 212–213
Self-regulation
    conceptualizations of, 15–16
    defined, 19
    documenting changes in, 113
    dynamic coaching approach
        additional resources, 82
        collaborative relationship building, 63–66
        context-based learning, 70–72
        instructing self-regulation, 72–78
        overview, 62
        structuring to model and facilitate self-regulation,
            66–70
        student benefits associated with, 79–82
    emotional, significance of, 18–19
    executive function problems and, 20–21
    executive functions and, 7, 15, 19, 21
    importance in high school and college, 19–20
    model of, 16–18

Self-regulation *(cont.)*
    outcomes, 114
    performance goals and, 110–112
Self-regulation goals
    in the development of a coaching plan, 114, 115,
        116–118
    overview and description of, 110–112
    pairing with performance goals in time management,
        168–170
    pairing with proximal goals, 117–118
    for self-advocacy, 201
    in self-learning, 162–163
Self-Regulation Skills Interview (SRSI), *100*
Semistructured interviews, 103–107, 113–114
"Sense of self"
    cognition and, 8
    metacognitive beliefs and, 16
Sensory/perceptual processes, *10*
Shell shock, 39
Sleep disorders, 40–41
SMARTER goals, 108–110
SMART goals, 108–109
Smartpens, 172, 186–187
Social relationships, challenges for military service
        members and veterans, 50
Social Support Questionnaire (SSQ), *100*, 114
Solution-based students, 66
Somatization, 41
Spaced retrieval, 71–72
Stages of change coaching model, 58–59, *60–61*
Story method strategy, *171*
Strategies
    managing ineffective strategies, 182–184
    for self-learning, 170–174
    for self-management, 174–182
    self-regulation and strategy plan implementation, 17
    in the self-regulation process, *74*, 75
    tracking in self-learning and self-management,
        184–186
Strategy Review and Other Applications (Form 4.8), 78,
        91, 213
Strategy Usefulness and Next Steps (Form 4.5), 77, 87,
        172, 186, 187, 203
Streaks ("habit tracker" app), 185
Stress, 46
Strides ("habit tracker" app), 185
Student Summary of Strategies (Form 4.7), 77, 90, 186, 187
Student Veterans of America (SVA), 47
Study guides, 161
Substance use, 42
Summarizing, in motivational interviewing, 64, *65*
Supplemental tests, for information gathering, 96–98
Support and instruction phase, *66*, 68–69
Support teams
    creating for self-advocacy, 201–203
    importance of, 66
    team approach to coaching self-advocacy, 199–201
Surveys, 98–107

TBI. *See* Traumatic brain injury
Team approach to coaching self-advocacy, 199–201
Team Members (Form 7.1), 200, 211
Templates for Goal Attainment Scaling (Form 5.9), 110,
        151–155
Test of Everyday Attention (TEA), *101*
Time management
    goal setting in, 166–170
    managing procrastination, 182–183
    strategizing for, 174–182
    in the support and instruction phase of coaching, 68
    systems employed by students, 168
    See also Self-management coaching
Time-management apps, 177–179
Total sleep deprivation, 41
Tracking
    of strategies and performance in self-learning and
        self-management, 184–186
    of strategy use for self-regulation, 76
Tracking Strategy Action (Form 4.4), 76, 86, 184–185, 186,
        187
Traumatic brain injury (TBI)
    college students with
        difficulties experienced by, 29–30
        enrollment at postsecondary institutions, 22, 23
        example of information gathering with, 95–96
        information gathering survey tools, 102–107
        student benefits associated with dynamic
            coaching, 80
    defined, 28
    executive function problems and, 29
    military service members and veterans with
        from blast exposure, 37–39
        effects on college performance, 48
        polytrauma clinical triad, 39
        trimorbid disorder, 42
    prevalence, 28–29
    See also Concussion
Trello (time-management app), *179*
Trimorbid disorder, 42

U.S. Department of Veterans Affairs, 53
U.S. Equal Employment Opportunity Commission, 195

VA. *See* U.S. Department of Veterans Affairs
VA Campus Toolkit, 54
Veterans. *See* Military service members and veterans
Veterans Crisis Line, 54
Veterans' organizations, 53
Visual imagery strategy, *171*
Visuospatial processes, *9*

War and the Soul (Tick), 42
Ways of Coping Questionnaire, *101*, 102
Wechsler Test of Adult Reading (WTAR), *101*
What to Expect with Dynamic Coaching (Form 4.1), 65, 83
Word-finding impairment, 164, 166
Working memory, 11